Successful Aging

Guest Editors

VINCENT MORELLI, MD
MOHAMAD SIDANI, MD

CLINICS IN
GERIATRIC MEDICINE

www.geriatric.theclinics.com

November 2011 • Volume 27 • Number 4

SAUNDERS an imprint of ELSEVIER, Inc.

W.B. SAUNDERS COMPANY
A Division of Elsevier Inc.

1600 John F. Kennedy Blvd., Suite 1800. Philadelphia, Pennsylvania 19103-2899

http://www.theclinics.com

CLINICS IN GERIATRIC MEDICINE Volume 27, Number 4
November 2011 ISSN 0749-0690, ISBN-13: 978-1-4557-0667-9

Editor: Yonah Korngold
Developmental Editor: Donald E. Mumford

Clinics in Geriatric Medicine (ISSN 0749-0690) is published quarterly by Elsevier Inc., 360 Park Avenue South, New York, NY 10010-1710. Months of issue are February, May, August, and November. Business and Editorial Offices: 1600 John F. Kennedy Blvd., Suite 1800, Philadelphia, PA 191023-2899. Periodicals postage paid at New York, NY, and additional mailing offices. Subscription prices is $241.00 per year (US individuals), $427.00 per year (US institutions), $167.00 per year (US student/resident), $314.00 per year (Canadian individuals), $532.00 per year (Canadian institutions), $333.00 per year (foreign individuals) and $532.00 per year (foreign institutions). Foreign air speed delivery is included in all *Clinics* subscription prices. All prices are subject to change without notice. POSTMASTER: Send address changes to *Clinics in Geriatric Medicine*, Elsevier Health Sciences Division, Subscription Customer Service, 3251 Riverport Lane, Maryland Heights, MO 63043. Telephone: 1-800-654-2452 (U.S. and Canada); 314-447-8871 (outside U.S. and Canada). Fax: 314-447-8029. E-mail: journalscustomerservice-usa@elsevier.com (for print support) or journalsonlinesupport-usa@elsevier.com (for online support).

Reprints. For copies of 100 or more, of articles in this publication, please contact the Commercial Reprints Department, Elsevier Inc., 360 Park Avenue South, New York, New York 10010-1710. Tel.: (212) 633-3812; Fax: (212) 462-1935, email: reprints@elsevier.com.

Clinics in Geriatric Medicine is covered in *MEDLINE/PubMed (Index Medicus), EMBASE/Excerpta Medica, Current Contents/Clinical Medicine (CC/CM),* and the *Cumulative Index to Nursing & Allied Health Literature.*

Printed and bound by CPI Group (UK) Ltd, Croydon, CR0 4YY
Transferred to Digital Print 2011

Contributors

GUEST EDITORS

VINCENT MORELLI, MD
Sports Medicine Fellowship Director, Department of Family and Community Medicine, Meharry Medical College, Nashville, Tennessee

MOHAMAD A. SIDANI, MD, MS
Associate Professor and Vice Chair for Clinical Affairs, Department of Family and Community Medicine, Meharry Medical College, Nashville, Tennessee

AUTHORS

NANA YAW ADU-SARKODIE, MD, MPH
Louisiana State University Health Sciences Center Geriatrics Fellowship, Kenner, Los Angeles

JERALYN ALLEN, MD
Sports Medicine Fellow, Department of Family and Community Medicine, Meharry Medical College, Nashville, Tennessee

JAMES CAMPBELL, MD
Associate Professor, Vice Chair and Director of Kenner Family Medicine Residency Program, Louisiana State University Health Sciences Center, Kenner, Los Angeles

CHARLES A. CEFALU, MD, MS
Professor and Chief, Section of Geriatric Medicine, Louisiana State University Health Sciences Center, New Orleans, Louisiana

GARY W. DUNCAN, MD
Professor and Interim Chair (Retired), Department of Neurology, Meharry Medical College, Nashville, Tennessee

ARTHUR T. FORT, MD
Assistant Professor of Family Medicine, Tulane University School of Medicine, New Orleans, Louisiana

KENT HOLTORF, MD
Holtorf Medical Group, Torrance, California

ASMA B. JAFRI, MD, MAcM
Clinical Professor, University of California, Riverside (UCR); and Assistant Clinical Professor, University of California Los Angeles (UCLA) Chair, Department of Family Medicine, Riverside County Regional Medical Center, Moreno Valley, California

COURTNEY J. KIHLBERG, MD, MSPH
Assistant Professor, Meharry Medical College, Department of Family and Community Medicine, Division of Preventive Medicine, Nashville, Tennessee

MICHELE M. LARZELERE, PhD
Assistant Professor, Family Medicine Residency, Louisiana State University Health Sciences Center, Kenner, Los Angeles

VINCENT MORELLI, MD
Sports Medicine Fellowship Director, Department of Family and Community Medicine, Meharry Medical College, Nashville, Tennessee

AROOB SHANAAH SALEH, MD
Fellow, Grant Medical Center Geriatric Fellowship Program, Columbus, Ohio

ERIKA SCHWARTZ, MD
Chief Medical Officer, Age Management Institute, New York, New York

MOHAMAD A. SIDANI, MD, MS
Associate Professor and Vice Chair for Clinical Affairs, Department of Family and Community Medicine, Meharry Medical College, Nashville, Tennessee

ROBERT SKULLY, MD
Program Director, Geriatric Fellowship; Associate Director, Grant Family Medicine Residency; Director, Acute Care for the Elderly Unit, Grant Medical Center; Clinical Assistant Professor, Ohio State University College of Medicine and Public Health, Columbus; Clinical Assistant Professor, Ohio University College of Osteopathic Medicine, Athens, Ohio

SARAH E. TAYLOR, DO
Chief Resident, Meharry Medical College, Department of Family and Community Medicine, Nashville, Tennessee

CAROL C. ZIEGLER, MS, RD, MSN, FNP
Instructor, Meharry Medical College, Department of Family and Community Medicine, Nashville, Tennessee

ROGER J. ZOOROB, MD, MPH, FAAFP
Professor, Meharry Medical College, Department of Family and Community Medicine, Nashville, Tennessee

Contents

Preface   xi

Vincent Morelli and Mohamad Sidani

Theories and Mechanisms of Aging   491

Charles A. Cefalu

This article discusses various theories of aging and their relative plausibility related to the human aging process. Structural and physiologic changes of aging are discussed in detail by organ system. Each of the organ systems is discussed when applicable to the various theories of aging. Normal versus abnormal aging is discussed in the context of specific aging processes, with atypical presentations of disease and general links to life expectancy. Life expectancy and life span are discussed in the context of advances in medical science and the potential ultimate link to human life span.

State of the Art in Anti-Aging Trends   507

Arthur T. Fort

This chapter is an effort to provide a cursory overview of current paradigms in the realm of anti-aging medicine. This subject will be evaluated according to current philosophic, clinical and scientific perspectives which are predominant in the field at this time.

Aging and Disease Prevention   523

Roger J. Zoorob, Courtney J. Kihlberg, and Sarah E. Taylor

This article reviews evidence-based recommendations for geriatric prevention disciplines and topics including health behaviors (eg, smoking cessation, physical activity), metabolic disorders, cardiovascular diseases, cancers, immunizations, depression, the promotion of independence, and polypharmacy. Recommendations for both the one-on-one, clinic-based setting and for community-wide initiatives are covered for each topic, as appropriate.

Hormone Replacement Therapy in the Geriatric Patient: Current State of the Evidence and Questions for the Future. Estrogen, Progesterone, Testosterone, and Thyroid Hormone Augmentation in Geriatric Clinical Practice: Part 1   541

Erika Schwartz and Kent Holtorf

This article presents an up-to-date review of the literature on hormone augmentation in the elderly to help primary care physicians better evaluate and utilize hormone replacement and optimization strategies to benefit their patients. The scientific literature suggests that hormone supplementation with estrogen, progesterone, testosterone, growth hormone, and thyroid hormone has the potential to improve quality of life and to prevent, or reverse, the many symptoms and conditions associated with aging, including fatigue, depression, weight gain, frailty, osteoporosis, loss of libido, and heart disease. Possible long-term side effects are also considered.

Hormone Replacement Therapy in the Geriatric Patient: Current State of the Evidence and Questions for the Future—Estrogen, Progesterone, Testosterone, and Thyroid Hormone Augmentation in Geriatric Clinical Practice: Part 2   561

Erika Schwartz, Vincent Morelli, and Kent Holtorf

The data reviewed herein show that hormone replacement therapies improve some conditions associated with aging. Additionally, some of the long-held fears of significant side effects associated with hormone supplementation may be overstated, especially when providing patients with individualized care and optimal monitoring. We encourage clinicians to consider such interventions based on the evidence presented. More long-term studies are needed to further quantify and substantiate the risks and benefits associated with the use of such therapies.

Diets for Successful Aging   577

Carol C. Ziegler and Mohamad A. Sidani

The effects of different dietary patterns on specific age-related illness and overall longevity are discussed.

Aging and the Effects of Vitamins and Supplements   591

Robert Skully and Aroob Shanaah Saleh

Vitamin supplements are commonly consumed by elderly patients. This article reviews the evidence behind vitamin supplementation in preventing disease states common in older age, with an emphasis on randomized controlled trials. In addition to vitamins, some commonly used supplements, such as ginkgo, DHEA, and omega-3 fatty acids, are also discussed.

Aging and Toxins   609

Asma B. Jafri

This article addresses physiologic organ system and cellular mechanisms of common toxic exposure in the elderly population. Air pollution, tobacco, alcohol, heat, cold, water pollution, medications, herbals, radiation, and other chemicals are discussed.

The Aging Brain and Neurodegenerative Diseases   629

Gary W. Duncan

> This article reviews the current thoughts on the effects of aging on the brain. Mechanisms of neurodegeneration are discussed, particularly those associated with Alzheimer's and Parkinson's diseases. Strategies of early detection of presymptomatic disease and potential future treatments are explored. Modification of risk factors and lifestyles for disease prevention is discussed.

Psychosocial Factors in Aging   645

Michele M. Larzelere, James Campbell, and Nana Yaw Adu-Sarkodie

> Many psychosocial factors have been associated with successful aging. The impact of social relationships, personality factors, self-perceptions, and religiosity/spirituality is reviewed in this article and recommendations for enhancing psychological aging are provided.

Aging and Exercise   661

Jeralyn Allen and Vincent Morelli

> In older adults, regular exercise provides numerous health benefits that include improvements in blood pressure, coronary artery disease, diabetes, lipid profile, osteoarthritis, osteoporosis, mood, neurocognitive function, and overall morbidity and mortality. This article discusses the benefits of exercise in the elderly and how physicians can help such patients overcome barriers to exercise (eg, sedentary lifestyle, lack of education, coexisting morbidities), and offers some practical exercise prescriptions for both healthy and compromised elderly patients.

Fatigue and Chronic Fatigue in the Elderly: Definitions, Diagnoses, and Treatments   673

Vincent Morelli

> Because fatigue is so prevalent in the elderly population, it is important that physicians be well versed in the evaluation and management of this complaint. This article discusses the clinical manifestations and predisposing factors for the three major categories of fatigue: recent, prolonged, and chronic. The CDC classification of chronic fatigue syndrome is included. Patient dissatisfaction with the care for their fatigue is a common problem. Several pharmaceutical treatment methods are presented. Non-pharmacologic options, such as use of vitamins, exercise, behavior modification, and diet are also discussed.

Toward a Comprehensive Differential Diagnosis and Clinical Approach to Fatigue in the Elderly   687

Vincent Morelli

> This article provides primary care physicians with an encompassing approach to fatigue to help generate a comprehensive differential diagnosis. Two-thirds of patients with fatigue will have an identifiable cause that can be elucidated with a careful history and appropriate laboratory tests. Accordingly, a wide range of differential diagnoses is presented.

Index   693

FORTHCOMING ISSUE

February 2012

Geriatric Oncology
Richard Rosenbluth, MD, *Guest Editor*

RECENT ISSUES

August 2011

Sarcopenia
Yves Rolland, MD, PhD, *Guest Editor*

May 2011

Update in the Medical Management of the
Long Term Care Patient
Miguel A. Paniagua, MD, *Guest Editor*

February 2011

Frailty
Jeremy D. Walston, MD, *Guest Editor*

Preface

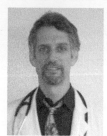
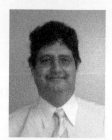

Vincent Morelli, MD   Mohamad Sidani, MD
Guest Editors

Research in the field of "successful aging" has increased dramatically in the last few decades. As a result, the public's awareness and interest in this area have been heightened. Today, more than ever, our patients are looking to us to serve as information analysts—to help them wade through the ever-rising sea of health information and misinformation that is widely distributed on the internet and available via the lay press.

This issue of *Clinics in Geriatric Medicine* will critically evaluate the literature in the rapidly changing field of "aging optimization medicine." As many primary care physicians begin to incorporate hormone therapy, exercise, diet, and other therapies into their practices, there is a need to separate scientific truth from wishful thinking. The ultimate goal is to understand the various risks and benefits involved with these therapies. Although many scientific studies have been performed in aging research in recent years, more remains to be done. Our aim is to separate what is known from what is hoped for, and to delineate the strengths, weaknesses, and limits of current medical literature. We hope that primary care providers and medical students will find our work well written, well researched, and clinically relevant.

We are pleased to serve as guest editors for this issue, and we feel privileged to have worked with such a distinguished group of collaborators. Many thanks to the contributing authors who have worked painstakingly to make their articles scholarly and relevant in the clinical setting. We also thank the Department of Family and Community Medicine at Meharry Medical College and the Family Medicine Department at Vanderbilt University Medical Center for providing us with the support needed to complete this project.

Clin Geriatr Med 27 (2011) xi–xii
doi:10.1016/j.cger.2011.07.014
0749-0690/11/$ – see front matter © 2011 Elsevier Inc. All rights reserved.

geriatric.theclinics.com

Thanks as well to the New Orleans Healing Center for their inspiration and direction. Finally, thanks to our editor at Elsevier, Barton Dudlick, without whose help this project would never have been accomplished.

Vincent Morelli, MD
Mohamad Sidani, MD
Department of Family and Community Medicine
Meharry Medical College
1005 Dr D.B. Todd Jr, Boulevard
Nashville, TN 37208-3599, USA

E-mail addresses:
vmorelli@mmc.edu (V. Morelli)
msidani@mmc.edu (M. Sidani)

Theories and Mechanisms of Aging

Charles A. Cefalu, MD, MS

KEYWORDS

- Aging • Telomeres • Free radicals
- Autoimmune theory of aging
- Genetic-developmental theory of aging

THEORIES OF AGING

Several theories may explain the normal aging process, either alone or in combination with other theories (**Table 1**). These theories can be generally classified into evolutionary, involving historical and evolutionary aspects of aging, and physiologic or structural and functional changes. Processes that may explain these theories at a cellular level include intrinsic timing mechanisms and signals, accidental chance events, programmed genetic signals making an organism more susceptible to accidental events, nuclear or mitochondrial DNA mutations or damage, damaged and abnormal proteins, cross-linkage, glycation, waste accumulation, general molecular wear and tear, free radical formation, and specific cellular components such as gene, chromosome, mitochondria, or telomeres. Physiologic processes that may explain aging include oxidative stress, immunologic, neuroendocrinologic, metabolic, and insulin signaling, and caloric restriction.[1]

The theory of oxidative stress has been popular over the last decade as extensive research has been performed evaluating the use of antioxidant vitamins such as B_{12}, folic acid, A, C, D, and E and their effect in slowing oxidative stress. It has been hypothesized that blocking free radical production as a result of oxidation and reduction through exposure of the human body to environmental toxins through excessive sunlight exposure (skin cancer), inhaled (lung cancer and chronic lung disease), and ingestion (carcinoma of the stomach or intestinal tract; macular degeneration and cataract; prostate cancer and Alzheimer's disease) may slow down the normal aging process. The theory is that highly reactive oxygen-derived substances (free radicals) result in the accumulation of protein, lipids, and DNA damage as a result of hypothermia and metabolism. It is postulated that reactive oxygen may be a signal for aging and its levels in tissues may determine the aging process and life span. Support for this theory is that mutations in the oxidative stress pathway may extend life span as evidenced by mutations of genes in other pathways that increase

Department of Medicine, Louisiana State University Health Sciences Center, 1542 Tulane Avenue, New Orleans, LA 70113, USA
E-mail address: ccefal@lsuhsc.edu

Clin Geriatr Med 27 (2011) 491–506
doi:10.1016/j.cger.2011.07.001
0749-0690/11/$ – see front matter © 2011 Elsevier Inc. All rights reserved.

geriatric.theclinics.com

Table 1
Major cellular and functional changes of aging by prominent theories and major associated clinical disease outcomes

Organ System	Major Theories	Cell Level	Structural/Functional Changes of Aging	Disease Outcomes
Integumentary	Oxidative stress; free radical; genetic; autoimmune	Melanocytes, mast, and Langerhans cells	Thinning of stratum corneum and subcutaneous layer	Squamous and basal cell carcinoma; malignant melanoma
Oral	Oxidative Stress; free radical; genetic; autoimmune	Buccal	Increased thickness of tooth dentin, decreased dental pulp; thinning of oral mucosa and receding of gums; decreased sensitivity for smell and taste	Squamous cell carcinoma; tooth decay
Visual	Oxidative stress; free radical; genetic	Rods and cones	Reduced night vision, accommodative ability and increased glare	Macular degeneration; cataracts; diabetic retinopathy
Hearing	Oxidative stress; free radical; genetic	Sensory and neural cells	Stiffening of the inner ear bones	Presbycusis; osteosclerosis
Musculoskeletal	Oxidative stress; genetic; autoimmune	Myocytes	Apoptosis, reduced size of myofibrils, decreased type 2 muscle fibers; decreased hand grip strength with more in the lower extremities	Falls; disuse atrophy; chronic musculoskeletal disorders
Skeletal	Oxidative stress; free radical; neuro endocrine	Osteoblasts and osteoclasts	Change in bone architecture and accumulation of microfractures, disparity in the concentration of deposited minerals, changes in the crystalline properties of mineral deposits and protein content of the matrix; decreased height and thinning of bone	Fractures

(continued on next page)

Table 1
(continued)

Organ System	Major Theories	Cell Level	Structural/Functional Changes of Aging	Disease Outcomes
Cardiovascular	Oxidative stress; free radical; neuroendocrine; genetic	Myocyte; pacemaker cell	Increase in left ventricular stiffness and decrease in compliance; decreased left ventricular diastolic filling and relaxation, increased stroke volume, reduction in maximal cardiac output and vasodilator response to exercise	Congestive heart failure; cardiomyopathy; heart block
Pulmonary	Oxidative stress; free radical; genetic; autoimmune	Alveolar cells	Chest wall stiffness; decreased arterial oxygenation and impaired carbon dioxide elimination; decrease in vital capacity and forced expiratory volume, increased residual volume and functional residual capacity	Chronic lung disease; carcinoma
Gastrointestinal	Oxidative stress; free radical	Mucosal cell	Decreased elasticity of connective tissue; reduction in phase I metabolism	Carcinoma; increased risk of drug–drug and drug–disease interactions
Renal/urogenital	Oxidative stress; free radical; genetic; neuroendocrine; autoimmune	Renal cell	Diminished proliferative reserve; apoptosis; loss of glomerular and tubular mass; decline in GFR, loss of tubular volume and narrowed homeostatic control of water and electrolyte balance	Carcinoma; chronic renal failure

(continued on next page)

Table 1
(continued)

Organ System	Major Theories	Cell Level	Structural/Functional Changes of Aging	Disease Outcomes
Neurologic	Oxidative stress; free radical; genetic; neuroendocrine	Neurons; glial cells	Decrease in size of hippocampus and frontal and temporal lobes; decreased number of receptors of all types in the brain with increased sensitivity; decrease in complex visuoconstructive skills and logical analysis skills; decrease in processing speed, decrease in reaction time and decrease ability to shift cognitive sets rapidly; memory distraction and decline in executive function; abnormal reflexes	Neuropathy; neurodegenerative disorders
Hematologic	Autoimmune; genetic; oxidative stress; free radical	Stem cells	Decreased marrow cellularity, increase in bone marrow fat and reduction in cancellous bone	Chronic anemia; myelofibrosis; leukemia
Neuroendocrine	Neuroendocrine; oxidative stress; genetic	Neuroendocrine cells; mitochondria	Decrease or increase in hormone levels; inability to conserve or dissipate heat	Autonomic neuropathy; thyroid disease; adrenal insufficiency; male and female menopause

longevity and exhibit enhanced resistance to stress and oxidative damage. However, most if not all research involving use of antioxidant vitamins to reduce oxidative stress have failed to yield positive results.[2]

Another theory of normal aging is related in part to the oxidative stress theory and is related to chromosomal alterations. Supposedly, deletions, mutations, translocations, and polyploidy are aged-acquired chromosomal instabilities that may contribute to gene silencing or expression of specific genes whose function are the production of specific cancers. Support for this theory is evidenced by research that indicates mitochondrial DNA mutations of genes in the oxidative stress pathway may contribute to reduced resistance to oxidative stress. However, such research showing significant impact on non-diseased aging is very small.[3]

Another popular theory of aging that has gained momentum in the last 10 years is the autoimmune theory that the human body essentially begins to produce autoantibodies to its own tissues and or the production of time-acquired deficits primarily in T-cell function predisposes the elderly to the development of infections, chronic disease, and cancer, particularly autoimmune diseases such as rheumatoid arthritis and systemic lupus erythematosis.[4]

The neuroendocrinologic theory proposes that cortisol surge or elevations related to chronic stress over the years may result in normal aging in the elderly's later years. Slower response to infections, age-related memory loss, reduced muscle function, and chronic inflammatory disease might be examples. It is hypothesized that a multimodal concept of controlling more effectively chronic inflammatory disease on a neuroendocrine–immune basis may reduce the normal aging process. However, research studies have failed to provide positive proof.[5]

Related to a fixed life span for humans, the developmental–genetic theory of aging related in part to the chromosomal alterations theory proposes that genetically programmed induction of senescence occurs which results in either the activation or suppression of specific "aging" genes. Support for this theory comes from studies that indicate that longevity in humans seems to be hereditable related to the presence of specific genes.[6] However, significant research showing that physical fitness also improves longevity in humans is somewhat counter to this theory, as is the theory of calorie restriction.

Calorie restriction and mutations in insulin-signaling pathways results in alterations in body size and composition, enhanced resistance to oxidative stress, and extended life span in a wide variety of species (yeasts, worms, flies, rodents). This has recently gained momentum as a very popular theory to explain normal aging in humans as significant research in these species has shown a correlation of calorie restriction with sarcopenia, cardiovascular disease, Alzheimer's disease, and cancer. One mechanism hypothesized is the stabilization of cell membranes, preventing functional decline in aging. However, research in humans is lacking.[7]

Telomeres are DNA sequences located at the ends of chromosomes and protect these ends. The telomere theory of aging postulates that normal somatic cells have a finite life span and lose telomeric DNA when they divide as a function of aging as noted in vitro studies. The telomerase enzyme adds telomere repeats to the ends of chromosomes. Critical shortening of the telomeric DNA owing to loss of the enzyme telomerase is the signal for the initiation of cellular senescence.[8] In vitro studies have also proven that reinstitution of telomerase and increase in length of the telomeric DNA resulted in extension of the cellular life span of human cells.[9]

ORGAN SYSTEM MECHANISMS OF AGING

The various organ system mechanisms of aging can be viewed in the context of both the cellular and clinical characteristics of normal aging that occur. Cellular changes with normal aging include decreased proliferative capacity and potential of specific cells (lymphocytes and fibroblasts) associated with decreased secretion of interleukin-2 and diminished expression of T-cell populations that have an altered affinity for this cytokine. The clinical characteristics of normal aging include a change in the biochemical composition of tissues (lipofuscin and extracellular matrix cross-linking, protein oxidation, and altered rates of gene transcription), reduction of physiologic capacity, reduced ability to maintain homeostasis (adaptive processes under physiologic stress), and increased susceptibility and vulnerability to disease. The various organ system mechanisms of aging are discussed in terms of specific structural and functional changes of normal aging.

Body Structure and Composition

Normal aging is associated with a reduction in height related to a decrease in the height of the vertebral body, thinning of the intervertebral discs, a certain amount of flexing of the hips and knees, and flattening of the arch of the foot. Normal patterns of weight loss are different for males and females by decade, but generally weight gain is seen until the age of 55 to 60 years, when decline begins. Weight changes with normal aging are affected by dietary habits, activity levels, culture, and economics. Fat and water content change with normal aging with lean body mass decreasing by 1% per year after age 55, with a reduction of 40% by age 80; fat composition doubles to 30% of total body weight by the seventh decade, and there is a greater increase possible in females.[10]

Balance and Gait

Normal changes in gait and balance include a reduction in gait velocities both for usual and maximal activity after the seventh decade. The gait is slower with shorter stride length and longer stance phase with both feet on the ground. There is also an impaired ability to stand longer on 1 foot, decreased power in the lower extremities, less ability to lean forward, and greater body sway when standing. Arm swing and plantar flexion are diminished. One of the consequences of these normal changes is an increased propensity to fall. Studies indicate that, with normal aging, a greater proportion of attentional resources are allocated to the balance demands of postural tasks to prevent falling.[11] Further, gait changes in older adults who walk with fear may be an appropriate response to unsteadiness, and are more likely a marker of underlying pathology, not simply a physiologic or psychological consequence of normal aging.[12]

Integumentary System

Changes of aging relative to the integumentary system can be further divided into intrinsic (physiologic) versus extrinsic (environmental) changes. Physiologic changes include structural changes, clinical manifestations of these changes, and physiologic and immunologic changes. Normal structural changes of aging of the integumentary system include a thinning of the stratum corneum, reduction in the number of Langerhans cells, melanocytes, and mast cells, and a reduction in the depth and extent of the subcutaneous fat layer. With these normal change and exposure to ultraviolet rays of the sun, structural changes of the skin may include decreased DNR repair and increased DNA injury, lysosomal damage, and altered collagen structure, resulting in an increased risk of skin cancer (basal cell, squamous cell, and melanoma). With normal aging, there is an increase in the proportion of hairs in the telogen or resting phase and shortening of the anagen or growth phase and a graying of hairs due to changes in the follicular melanocytes.

An end result of these structural changes is varying degrees of thinning of the hair or actual balding; to some extent, this is related to genetic predisposition. Other clinical changes related to these structural changes include an increased frequency of benign and malignant epidermal neoplasms, irregular pigmentation, a propensity to blister formation, a reduction of dermal clearance of chemical agents leading to dermatitis and slower healing, superficial skin laxity, increased risk of skin tears, and thermoregulatory disturbances such as hypothermia and hyperthermia. Functional normal changes of the skin include beta cell dysfunction and increased levels of immunoglobulins A and G and a reduction in epidermal 7 dehydrocholesterol per unit area, resulting in a reduction in subsequent vitamin D production in the skin. This may result in an increased frequency of clinical disease including increased frequency of antigen–antibody reactions, increased risk of skin infection, and development of osteomalacia and fracture.[13]

Oral, Dental, Vision, Hearing, and Olfactory Systems

Normal dental changes of aging include increased thickness of the tooth dentin, diminished volume of the dental pulp, and a shift in the proportion of nervous, vascular, and connective tissues. As a result, there is an increased risk of dental infection, increased risk of tooth brittleness, increased sensitivity to irritants, and diminished reparative capacity. Normal oral changes of aging include thinning of the oral mucosa with receding of the gums and a reduction in the amount of lingual papillae. The end result is an increased risk of plaque formation, inflammation, and infection, as well as a decreased ability to detect salt, bitter, sweet, and sour. Although atrophy of the alveolar bone occurs with normal aging, the process is accelerated in the process of osteoporosis. Coupled with tooth decay over time, this may lead to tooth loss and need for dentures when excessive.[14]

Normal vision changes with aging include presbyopia, reduced contrast sensitivity, impaired adaptation to darkness or light, and delayed recovery time to glare. There is also reduced papillary size and yellowing and opacification of the lens. These changes result in normal clinical vision changes associated with aging and include reduced night vision, increased glare, and reduced accommodative ability of the pupils. There is greater difficulty identifying objects in shadows or adjusting to dark with scattering of light leading to glare sensitivity. Older individuals require brighter light that is free from glare. Coupled with older individuals' increased response time to acute situations, this has implications for the older driver and these individuals should limit their driving to short distances, only during daytime hours, and during low traffic volume periods.[15,16]

With normal aging, progressive damage to sensory cells and neurons of the inner ear may occur owing to ototoxic drugs, physical stimulation (excitotoxins, loud noises), free radicals, the removal of growth factors, and even normal aging. There also seems to be stiffening of the middle ear bones, resulting in reduced elasticity and increased frequency of otosclerosis. The end result over time with advancing age may be decreased ability to discriminate words or sounds and an increased frequency of high-pitch, high-frequency hearing loss (presbycusis). Appropriate communication techniques for the affected senior include face-to-face interaction (for lip reading), a room free of background noise, and speaking in a slow and low tone voice.[17,18] There is also reduced function of the olfactory nerve and reduced sensitivity of the taste buds in the oral cavity, resulting in reduced sensation of smell and taste. Clinically, this may result in reduced appetite and progressive weight loss leading to malnutrition in the oldest old, including those with dementia and or depression. Use of liberalized diets with taste enhancers may improve appetite and quality of life for these patients.[19]

Musculoskeletal System

During normal aging, there is a significant loss of skeletal mass that can have a dramatic impact on the quality of life of the older adult. This muscle loss primarily involves type 2 fibers where there is a decrease in size and or number of myofibrils and altered innervations of these myofibrils. It is hypothesized that, at the mitochondrial level, there is superoxide generation at complexes I and III of the electron transport chain.[20] Normal aging is associated with apoptosis as a mechanism of loss of muscle cells in and plays an important role in age-related sarcopenia.[21] Normal functional changes in the musculoskeletal system include a significant reduction in hand grip strength with the loss being greater in the lower than in the upper extremities.

Peak bone density is achieved in the 30s and is then accompanied by a 1% and 0.7% resorption in females and males, respectively, per year.[22] Bone formation and resorption may vary from 1 older adult to another depending on vitamin D, estrogen, and testosterone levels. Normal changes in bone are both qualitative and quantitative, and include alterations in the dynamics of bone cell populations, changes in bone architecture, accumulation of microfractures, disparity in the concentration of deposited minerals, changes in the crystalline properties of mineral deposits, and changes in the protein content of matrix material.[23] With normal aging, there is a decline in cortical thickness of the vertebrae and a disruption of the trabecular network resulting in a 4- to 6-fold decrease in vertebral strength and a 2- to 4-fold increase in the risk of vertebral fragility fractures of the spine.[24] Joints become stiffer owing to a reduction in water content in the tendons, ligaments, cartilage, and synovial compartments. Related to this is an increase in keratin sulfate and hyaluronic acid content of cartilage.[25] Connective tissues become stiffer with normal aging, which can be modified by physical exercise. In addition, the chemical–physical stability of collagen is a precise measure for the functional age of the individual. It is hypothesized that shortening of the telomeres with accelerated aging is associated with the development of disease states related to collagen production such as segmental progeroid syndromes (dyskeratosis congenita).[26]

The Cardiovascular System

Normal changes of aging of the cardiovascular system are both structural and functional. There is a progressive loss of and hypertrophy of myocytes. There is also a loss of 90% of the pacemaker cells in the sinus node by the age of 75 years, resulting in slower resting and maximum heart rates, and that related to activity or exertion. Maximum left ventricular stiffness increases with a decrease in compliance. When coupled with a reduced and maximal heart rate, the heart compensates by increasing stroke volume with a reduction in maximal cardiac output and vasodilator response to exercise. There is also decreased left ventricular diastolic filling and relaxation, which is compensated for by a contribution from left atrial contraction. Owing in part to calcification of the vessel walls, increase in diameter, loss of compliance resulting from collagen deposition, and fragmentation of elastin of the central and peripheral vascular system, there is increased systemic vascular resistance.[27] The responses to parasympathetic withdrawal as well as sympathetic stimulation decline with age, and both of these factors contribute to the reduced cardiovascular responses to stress with advancing age.[28] As a result, there is an increased risk of congestive heart failure or heart block in the presence of long-standing disease processes such as diabetes, hypertension, or coronary artery disease.

A common but often overlooked clinical finding in the oldest old or those over the age of 85 is the finding of a wide pulse pressure with a high systolic and low diastolic or Osler's hypertension (pseudohypertension). Documentation of Osler's hypertension involves inflating the blood pressure cuff and listening for the pulsating sounds in the antecubital area with the stethoscope. Osler's hypertension is present if the radial or antecubital artery is palpable after the pulsatile sounds by stethoscope go away with inflation of blood pressure cuff.[29] Caution should be advised in the overtreatment of this clinical state by treating the high systolic greater than 160 mmHg at the risk of lowering the diastolic to dangerously low levels (<80 or <70) because this could increase the risk of hypoperfusion and subsequent development of stroke, heart failure, renal failure, or myocardial infarction. On the other hand, 10% to 15% of older normal individuals may have postural hypotension defined as a drop in systolic blood pressure of 20 mmHg on standing or sitting from a lying position. This may be because of blunted baroreceptors in the carotid arteries with normal aging that do not sense acute changes in blood pressure on position change and therefore associated with a blunted heart rate increase to balance the drop in pressure.[30]

Pulmonary System

The respiratory system undergoes various immunologic, structural, and physiologic changes with normal aging. Structural changes of aging of the pulmonary system include chest wall and thoracic spine deformities, alterations in the connective tissue, reduced size of the airways, and shallower alveolar cells and sacs. The lung parenchyma loses its supporting structure, causing dilation of air spaces. There is a 25% reduction in diaphragmatic strength of the intercostals muscles encompassing the rib cage due to sarcopenia and muscle atrophy.[31] This can also impair cough, which is critical for airway clearance. These normal changes may increase the risk of pneumonia in the presence of chronic neurologic or muscle disease (multiple sclerosis, cerebrovascular accident, Parkinson's disease).

After age 20 to 25 years and thereafter with normal aging, there is a progressive decline in lung function. With the increase in alveolar dead space with normal aging, arterial oxygen is affected without impairing carbon dioxide elimination. Other functional pulmonary changes associated with normal aging include a decline of vital capacity and forced expiratory volume in 1 second of 25 to 30 mL per year after age 65. There is also an increase in residual volume and functional residual capacity. The normal oxygen gradient through the pulmonary alveolus is increased with age and the blood oxygen saturation decreases with age by the formula, Pao_2 (blood oxygenation level percent) $= 110 - (0.4 \times age)$. The airway receptors undergo functional changes with normal aging and are less likely to respond to drugs in the same fashion as younger patients. In addition, normal aging is associated with a decreased sensation of dyspnea and reduced ventilator response to hypoxia and hypercapnea, increasing the risk of ventilator failure during periods of high demand states, such as heart failure and pneumonia, and possibly resulting in poor outcomes.[32] In addition, an abnormal inflammatory response in the lungs from inhaled particles and gases (usually from cigarette smoke) is considered to be the general pathogenic mechanism for the development of chronic obstructive pulmonary disease. An important component of this inflammation seems to be activation of leukocytes and development of oxidant–antioxidant and protease–anti-protease imbalances.[33]

Gastrointestinal System

Structural and functional changes of the gastrointestinal system are multiple and are to some extent secondary to the physiologic changes of aging. Structural changes in connective tissue that limit the elasticity of the gastrointestinal tract and alterations in nerves and muscles result in impaired motility. In the stomach, distensibility decreases and early satiety occurs as a result, although gastric emptying time and acid production are not affected. There is a decrease in motility in the large intestine resulting in an increased frequency of constipation with normal aging. There is a tendency to develop diverticulosis owing to stretching laxity of the arterial muscular rings as they enter the colon mucosa and elevated pressure in the colon owing to straining. In the small intestine, transit time is not affected, but absorption of calcium and vitamin D is impaired. There is a decrease in liver size, mass, and blood flow. Pancreas exocrine or endocrine function is not affected, but the pancreas is displaced inferiorly.[34]

Physiologically, there is a reduction in phase I (oxidation and reduction) but no change in phase II (acetylation, methylation, and sulfation) metabolism. This has implications for the dosage and use of specific pharmacologic agents in the elderly. Agents such as diazepam, diazepoxide, and flurazepam are long acting benzodiazepines and must be metabolized by phase I. Therefore, their levels are likely to be increased excessively and on a prolonged basis, contributing to sedation, falls, cognitive dysfunction, and even depression. These agents are specifically contraindicated in the elderly. Other agents that must be metabolized include the barbiturates, nonsteroidal inflammatory drugs, aspirin, calcium channel blockers, acetaminophen, α-blockers, erythromycin, statins, ketoconazole, phenytoin, tetracyclines, valproic acid, lidocaine, carbamazepine, metoprolol, tricyclic antidepressants, selective serotonin reuptake inhibitors, and neuroleptics. They should be used with caution in the elderly, with a reduction in dosage and careful monitoring. Amitriptyline, fluoxetine, and barbiturates are also contraindicated in the elderly because of their high anticholinergic activity (falls, hypotension, lethargy) and long half-life (nausea, decreased appetite).[35]

Renal System

With normal aging, the renal system is associated with structural and physiologic changes of aging. Cellular changes with normal aging include a diminished proliferative reserve, an increased tendency to apoptosis, alterations in growth factor profiles, and changes in potential progenitor and immune cell functions.[36] Structural changes include a loss of glomerular and tubular mass. Renal function as measured by glomerular filtration rate (GFR) declines after age 40 at a mean rate of 1% per year and accelerating in the later years in two thirds of older individuals. However, because the Baltimore Longitudinal Study indicated that a decline in GFR did not occur in one half of study participants, a decline in kidney function is not inevitable. There is also a reduced GFR, loss of tubular volume, and narrowed homeostatic control of water and electrolyte balance. Despite these significant structural and physiologic changes, the normal aging kidney is able to maintain homeostasis of body fluids and electrolytes in most cases, except in the presence of environmental and disease-related stresses (volume changes or alterations in acid–base balance) when the aging kidney is slower to respond with diuresis or conservation of fluid volume, resulting in an increased risk of hypervolemia and hypovolemia. However, the aging kidney has reduced ability to secrete sodium.[37,38] There is evidence that oxidant stress and inflammation at the cellular level may result in these normal cellular changes and in excess may lead to chronic kidney disease.[39]

Physiologic changes of the normal kidney have significant implications for drugs mostly eliminated by the kidneys. Common classes of drugs for which dosage reduction is prudent to prevent side effects includes fluroquinolones (phototoxicity, hallucinations, delusions, seizures, cognitive dysfunction), aminoglycosides (kidney failure, hearing loss, tinnitus), penicillins (seizures, cognitive dysfunction), digoxin (reduced appetite, nausea, depression, visual problems), and H2 blockers (confusion and cognitive dysfunction), angiotensin-converting enzyme inhibitors (worsening renal failure), metformin (contraindicated if GFR is ≤35 mL), bisphosphonates (contraindicated if GFR is <30 mL), and thiazides (may not be effective and risk of dehydration). Other classes of drugs primarily eliminated by the kidney in which dosage should be reduced include procainamide, atenolol, clofibrate, lithium, and fluconazole.

Urogenital System

Normal changes of the urogenital system are structural and physiologic. Structurally in the male, there is increased size of the prostate; in the older female, there is an increased frequency of decreased vaginal lubrication or dryness, and thinning of the vaginal mucosa. Physiologically, there is an elevation of the prostate-specific antigen with advanced age per decade related to the increased mass or density of the prostate. Follicle-stimulating hormone and luteinizing hormone levels also increase during the perimenopausal period and thereafter. Asymptomatic bacteruria is a common phenomenon seen with advancing age owing to reflux of bacteria from the vaginal vault or from prostatic hyperplasia and the presence of laxity of the urethra with aging. Functionally, 10% to 15% of older, normal individuals may have detrusor hyperactivity resulting in urinary frequency. Coupled with reduced immune defense mechanisms with normal aging in the advanced elderly, there is a greater risk for urinary tract infection in the absence of structural deficits of the urogenital tract.[40]

The Nervous System

Structural changes of the central nervous system with normal aging include a decrease in the size of the hippocampus and the frontal and temporal lobes. Structurally, there is also a decreased number of receptors of all types in the brain; the remaining receptors are more sensitive so that the same dosage of central acting pharmacologic agents are likely to have an exaggerated effect resulting in sedation, cognitive dysfunction, or drowsiness and resulting in an increased frequency of adverse drug reactions. Physiologically, there is evidence that oxidative stress and the accumulation of nitric oxide and mutations and deletions of DNA may play a role in Alzheimer's disease and other neurodegenerative diseases of aging.[41,42] Normal functional changes of the brain also include a decrease in short-term memory for recent events and encoding and retrieval is decreased. Complex visuoconstructive skills and logical analysis skills decrease. There is a decrease in overall processing speed, less ability to shift cognitive sets rapidly, and a decrease in reaction time. Memory is also more susceptible to distraction and problems develop with novel tasks that require quick psychomotor responses. Most cognitive decline occurs in executive function and not memory.[43,44] Subtle neurologic abnormalities may be detected on a normal neurologic examination of an older patients, including diminished arm swing, diminished toe vibration sense, hyperreflexia in the arms, unequal nasolabial folds, absent papillary response, Babinski sign, diminished position sense, and diminished arm strength. There are also changes in the sleep pattern of older normal individuals. These include less total time in stage III and IV sleep cycles and more time in stage I and II non-rapid eye movement sleep. Older individuals also spend more time awake in bed, have more frequent awakenings during the night, experience a greater period of sleep latency before going to sleep, and have less total sleep time.[45]

Autoregulation and Neuroendocrine Function

At the cellular level, cells count on precise mechanisms that regulate protein homeostasis to maintain a functional and stable proteome.[46] With both normal aging, proteasome inhibition alters specific aspects of neural mitochondrial homeostasis and also alters lysosomal-mediated degradation of mitochondria. This inhibition may also lead to aged-related disease in the nervous system.[47] In addition, the accumulation of various physiologic and psychological stressors may have a significant impact on the nervous, endocrine, and immune systems with normal aging associated with age-related disease.[48] Aberrant insulin receptor signaling and amino acid homeostasis causing oxidative stress may also play a role.[49] Physiologically, normal aging is associated with lower estrogen, testosterone, thyroid-stimulating hormone, and DHEA-S levels, as well as increased prolactin levels.[50] Functionally, with advanced aging, these physiologic changes with normal aging may be associated with an inability to conserve or dissipate heat efficiently. When faced with very cold temperatures, the older individual may not be able to conserve body heat quickly enough to prevent the development of hypothermia. Likewise, when faced with extremely hot weather, the older individual may not be able to dissipate heat quickly enough to prevent heat exhaustion or stroke. In part, this is because of a reduction in the elasticity of the vascular system, as discussed.

Hematopoietic System

Structural and functional changes of the hematopoietic system occur with aging both at the microscopic and macroscopic levels. At the microscopic level, bone marrow cellularity decreases to about 50% after 30 years followed by a further decline to 30% after age 65. This reduction may be related to an increase in bone marrow fat and a reduction in the volume of cancellous (spongy) bone, but is unrelated to a decrease in hematopoietic tissue. Telomere shortening, a determinant of the number of divisions a cell undergoes, has not been shown to be associated with age-related bone marrow stem cell exhaustion. However, when subjected to stress, there is diminished self-renewal capacity, restriction of the breadth of developmental potency, and decreased numbers of progeny of old stem cells subjected to hematopoietic demands. There is considerable debate as to whether published normal ranges for hemoglobin, hematocrit, and other hematologic indices are the same in older as in younger adults, because normal aging is accompanied by physiologic changes and the subsequent progression of disease.[51,52] Structural changes include an increased amount of iron stores in the bone marrow and replacement of fibrous tissue in the bone marrow itself, resulting in a certain degree of myelofibrosis.

NORMAL VERSUS AGING AND SUCCESSFUL VERSUS USUAL AGING

There is confusion as to what is normal and what constitutes disease, especially as it related to particular disease processes. New research findings continuously refine the concept of normal aging versus disease as it relates to specific disease processes. Anemia has been discussed. Normal aging of the kidney versus renal disease is another example. Depending on what formula is used determines at what point an individual may have renal disease.[53] Another example involves the issue of osteoporosis. The medical literature defines osteopenia as bone mineral density between 1.0 and 2.5 SD below that of a "young normal" adult (T-score between −1.0 and −2.5) and normal bone as bone mineral density within 1 SD of a "young normal" adult (T-score at −1.0 and above).[54] However, for a specific older individual, that cutpoint may not specifically describe that person's bone status when various factors come into play (diet, exercise, calcium, and vitamin D intake, in addition to genetics). It is anticipated that further research will reveal the answers to these and other questions.

Experts in the field of aging also believe that there is a distinct difference between successful versus usual aging and that it has an impact on life expectancy and quality of life. Successful aging involves the practice of primary and to a lesser extent secondary prevention.[55] Examples of primary prevention include regular mental and physical exercise; caloric restriction, weight loss, and regular consumption of fruits and vegetables, nuts, and whole wheat products; smoking prevention and cessation; limited exposure to environmental toxins (second-hand smoke, pollution, sun exposure) and chemical free radicals (high fat intake); multivitamin supplementation; and regular vaccination (influenza, pneumonia, zoster; diphtheria/tetanus). Secondary prevention involves prevention of secondary disease: control of hypertension and daily aspirin consumption (81mg); control of diabetes or other chronic illness; reduction in cholesterol and triglyceride levels; and regular medical follow-up.[56]

Regular exercise in normal older individuals has been shown to have multiple beneficial effects, including reduction in fall risk, stabilization of or improved cognition, improvement in mood and emotional well-being, and reduction in cardiovascular morbidity (myocardial infarction, cerebrovascular accident, peripheral vascular disease).[57]

LIFE SPAN AND LIFE EXPECTANCY

Life span for humans is said to be fixed as is the case for other species. However, life expectancy has increased over the last 50 to 75 years owing to advances in medical technology and research. Examples include the discovery of penicillin and the antibiotic era and with a significant increase in life expectancy related to prevention of death from pneumonia and tuberculosis through the development of a comprehensive and exhaustive list of antibiotics and anti-tuberculous agents. In the cardiovascular era, the incidence of stroke, kidney failure, congestive heart failure, and myocardial infarction was reduced with the use of newer anti-hypertensives, aspirin, and cholesterol-reducing agents. In biotechnology and immunology era, the incidence or progression of cancer has been reduced with the use of biotechnology and immunologic agents. And yet to be determined is the effect that environmental pollutants will have on the delineation between normal aging versus disease and subsequent life expectancy as new laws are passed in the United States to improve the quality of the air and reduce the ingestion of foods with potentially harmful additives (insecticides, hormones, preservatives, and antibiotics).[58] And then there is the controversial issue of using stem cell research to prevent or reverse disease, with the potential ethical implications related to cloning and genetic engineering. It is conceivable that stem cell research may also reveal other mysteries of aging that may ultimately expand life span and are now considered to be normal changes of aging, but in the future may actually represent preventable disease.

REFERENCES

1. Pacala JT, Sullivan Gm. Geriatric review syllabus: a core curriculum in geriatric medicine. 7th edition. New York: American Geriatrics Society; 2010. p. 9–14.
2. Zasshi Y. Analysis of Aging-related oxidative stress status in normal aging animals and development of anti-aging interventions. Yakugaku Zasshi 2010;130:29–42.
3. Lucas JN, Deng W, Moore D, et al. Background ionizing radiation plays a minor role in the production of chromosome translocations in a control population. Int J Radiat Biol 1999;75:819–27.
4. Kent S. Can normal aging be explained by the immunologic theory. Geriatrics 1997;32:111–6.
5. Weinert BT, Timiras PS. Invited review: theories of aging. J Appl Physiol 2003;95: 1706–16.
6. Lagaay AM, D'Amaro J, Ligthart GJ, et al. Longevity and heredity in humans. Association with the human leucocyte antigen phenotype. Ann N Y Acad Sci 1991; 621:78–89.
7. YU BP, Morgan TE, Wong AM, et al. Anti-inflammatory mechanisms of dietary restriction in slowing aging processes. Interdiscip Top Gerontol 2007;35:83–97.
8. Artandi SE. Telomeres, telomerase, and human disease. N Engl J Med 2006;355: 1195–7.
9. Vaziri H, Benchimol S. Reconstitution of telomerase activity in normal human cells leads to elongation of telomeres and extended replicative life span. Curr Biol 1998;8: 279–82.
10. Dharmarajan TS, Ugalino JT. The physiology of aging. In: Dharmarajan TS, Norman RA, editors. Clinical geriatrics. Boca Raton (FL): The Parthenon Publishing Group; 2003. p. 9–22.
11. Lajoie Y, Teasdale N, Bard C, et al. Upright standing and gait: are there changes in atttentional requirements related to normal aging? Exp Aging Res 1996;22:185–98.
12. Herman T, Giladi N, Gurevich T, et al. Gait Instability and fractal dynamics of older adults with a "cautious" gait: why do certain older adults walk fearfully? Gait Posture 2005;21:178–85.
13. Cefalu CA, Nesbitt L. Common dermatological conditions in aging. In: Rosenthal T, Naughton B, Williams M, editors. Office care geriatrics. Philadelphia: Lippincott Williams & Wilkins; 2006. p. 491–2.
14. Pacala JT, Sullivan Gm. Geriatric review syllabus: a core curriculum in geriatric medicine, 7th edition. New York: American Geriatrics Society; 2010. p. 390–1.
15. Sloane PD. Normal aging. In: Harm RJ, Sloane PD, Warshaw GA, editors. Primary care geriatrics, 5th edition. St. Louis: Mosby; 2002. p. 23–4.
16. Buch ER, Young S, Contreras-Vidal JL. Visuomotor adaptation in normal aging. Learn Mem 2003;10:55–63.
17. Waters C. Molecular mechanisms of cell death in the ear. Ann N Y Acad Sci 1999;884:41–51.
18. Caspary DM. Aging and hearing. Hear Res 2010;264:1–2.
19. Position of the American dietetic Association. Liberalization of the diet prescription improves quality of life for older adults in long-term care. J Am Diet Assoc 2005;105: 1955–65.
20. Jackson MJ. Skeletal muscle aging: role of reactive oxygen species. Crit Care Med 2009;37(10 Suppl):S368–71.
21. Braga M, Sinha Hikim AP, Datta S, et al. Involvement of oxidative stress and caspase 2-mediated intrinsic pathway signaling in age-related increase in muscle cell apoptosis in mice. Apoptosis 2008;13:822–32.

22. O'Flaherty EJ. Modeling normal aging bone loss, with consideration of bone loss in osteoporosis. Toxicol Sci 2000;55:171–88.
23. Kiebzak Gm. Age-related bone changes. Exp Gerontol 1991;26:171–87.
24. Mosekilde L. Vertebral structure and strength in vivo and in vitro. Calcif Tissue Int 1993;53(Suppl 1):S121–5.
25. Hofer AC, Tran RT, Aziz OZ, et al. Shared phenotypes among segmental progeroid syndromes suggest underling pathways of aging. J Gerontol A Biol Sci Med Sci 2005;60:10–20.
26. Pugh KG, Wei JY. Clinical implications of physiological changes in the aging heart. Drugs Aging 2001;18:263–76.
27. Stratton JR, Levy WC, Caldwell JH, et al. Effects of aging on cardiovascular responses to parasympathetic withdrawal. J Am Coll Cardiol 2003;41:2077–83.
28. Cheng TO. Osler maneuver to detect pseudohypertension. JAMA 1999;282:943.
29. Mader SL. Aging and postural hypotension. An update. J Am Geriatr Soc 1989;37: 129–37.
30. Tolep K, Higgins N, Muza S, et al. Comparison of diaphragm strength between healthy adult elderly and young men. Am J Respir Crit Care Med 1995;152:677–82.
31. Sharma G, Goodwin James. Effects of aging on respiratory system physiology and immunology. Clin Intervent Aging 2006;1:253–60.
32. MacNee W. Accelerated lung aging: a novel pathogenic mechanism of chronic obstructive pulmonary disease. Biochem Soc Trans 2009;37:819–23.
33. Altman DF. Changes in gastrointestinal, pancreatic, biliary, and hepatic function with aging. Gastroenterol Clin North Am 1990;19:227–34.
34. Cefalu CA. Clinical pharmacology. In: Burke M, Laramie JA, editors. Primary care of the older adult: a multidisciplinary approach. 2nd edition. St. Louis: Mosby; 91–154.
35. Schmitt R, Cantley LG. The impact of aging on kidney repair. Am J Physiol Renal Physiol 2008;294:F1265–72.
36. Rainfray M, Richard-Harston S, Salles-Montaudon N, et al. Effects of aging on kidney function and implications for medical practice. Presse Med 2000;29:1373–8.
37. Beck LH. The aging kidney. Defending a delicate balance of fluid and electrolytes. Geriatrics 2000;55:26–8.
38. Vlassera H, Torreggiani M, Post JB, et al. Role of oxidants, inflammation in declining renal function in chronic kidney disease and normal aging. Kidney Int Suppl 2009; 114:S3–11.
39. Cefalu CA. Urinary incontinence. In: Ham RJ, Sloan PJ, Warshaw G, et al, editors. Primary care geriatrics. 5th edition. New York: Mosby/Elsevier; 2007. p. 306–23.
40. Filipcik P, Cente M, Ferencik M, et al. The role of oxidative stress in the pathogenesis of Alzheimer's disease. Bratislavske Lekarske Listy 2006;107:384–94.
41. Rao KS. Free radical induced oxidative damage in DNA: relation to brain aging and neurological disorders. Indian J Biochem Biophys 2009;46:9–15.
42. Weiner MF, Lipton Am. Alzheimer's disease and other dementias. Washington (DC): American Psychiatric Publishing, Inc.; 2009.
43. Sadavpu K. et al. Comprehensive textbook of geriatric psychiatry, 3rd edition. New York: WW Norton and Co; 2004.
44. Vaz Fragoso CA, Gill TM. Sleep complaints in community-living older persons: a multifactorial geriatric syndrome. J Am Geriatr Soc 2007;55:1853–66.
45. Morimoto RI, Cuervo AM. Protein homeostasis and aging: taking care of proteins from the cradle to the grave. J Gerontol A Biol Sci Med Sci 2009;64:167–70.
46. Sullivan PG, Dragicevic NB, Deng JH, et al. Proteasome inhibition alters neural mitochondrial homeostasis and mitochondria turnover. J Biol Chem 2004;279: 20699–707.

47. Pederson WA, Wan R, Mattson MP. Impact of aging on stress-responsive neuro endocrine systems. Mech Ageing Dev 2001;122:963–83.
48. Drage W, Kinscherf R. Aberrant insulin receptor signaling and amino acid homeostasis as a major cause of oxidative stress in aging. Antiox Redox Signal 2008; 10:661–78.
49. Salvini S, Stampfer MJ, Barbieri RL, et al. Effects of age, smoking and vitamins on plasma DHEAS levels: a cross-sectional study in men. J Clin Endocrinol Metab 1992;74:139–43.
50. Rodak BF, Fritsma GA, Doig K. Pediatric and geriatric hematology. In: Hematology: clinical principles and applications. 3rd edition. St. Louis: Elsevier; 2007. p. 531.
51. Van Zant G, Liang Y. The role of stem cells in aging. Exp Hematol 2003;31:659–72.
52. Heras M, Guerrero MT, Fernandez-Reyes MJ, et al. Estimation of glomerular filtration rate in persons aged 68 years or older: agreement between distinct calculation methods. Rev Esp Geriatr Gerontol 2010;45:86–8.
53. National Osteoporosis Foundation. Clinical guide to prevention and treatment of osteoporosis. Available at: http://www.nof.org/sites/default/files/pdfs/NOF_ClinicianGuide2009_v7.pdf. Accessed July 7, 2011.
54. Inelmen EM, Sergi G, Enzi G, et al. New approach to gerontology: building up "successful aging" conditions. Aging Clin Exp Res 2007;19:160–4.
55. US Preventive Health Task Force. Clinical practice guidelines. Available at: http://www.ahrq.gov/clinic/cpgsix.htm. Accessed July 7, 2011.
56. Nusselder WJ, Franco OH, Peeters A, et al. Living healthier for longer: comparative effects of three heart healthy behaviors on life expectancy with and without cardiovascular disease. BMC Public Health 2009;9:487.
57. Tosato M, Zamboni V, Ferrini A, et al. The aging process and potential interventions to extend life expectancy. Clin Intervent Aging 2007;2:401–12.

State of the Art in Anti-Aging Trends

Arthur T. Fort, MD

KEYWORDS

• Elderly • Anti-aging • Calorie-restriction • Gerontology

A text on successful aging would be incomplete without a discussion of what may, or potentially will, be done to retard, delay and, in general, avoid the pitfalls of aging. This has been a universal human pursuit as far back as we have been sentient and, at this time, science may actually be making some reasoned progress in this direction. Research is now offering real hope in extending lifespan in both qualitative and quantitative terms. Scientific inquiry in aging is growing almost exponentially. For example, a Pubmed search for resveratrol returns 3,751 different papers, while a search for anti-aging medicine returns 1,989 results.

There are numerous, well-funded anti-aging research centers populated with first rate scientists running at full tilt. The National Institute of Aging is among them. The National Institute of Aging has a program known as the "Interventions Testing Program," which selects and evaluates a handful of promising anti-aging compounds annually. The equivalent testing of each substance chosen occurs in 3 different independent laboratories to verify that all of the results are accurate and replicable. With this system, promising compounds are rapidly and systematically ruled in or out for future research. The pursuit of anti-aging research is unquestionably established and moving forward rapidly.

The pharmaceutical industry is involved in anti-aging more indirectly. The US Food and Drug Administration (FDA) does not classify aging as a disease; thus, it is not possible to have the appropriate trials for FDA approval, even if a drug was available that could be shown to extend maximum human lifespan. Because of this, drug companies seek pharmaceuticals which alleviate aspects of aging and, if it turns out they might extend maximum lifespan, that would be a nice bonus. Pursuing drugs that extend lifespan is generally consistent with drugs that inhibit or reverse diseases of aging, so the obstacle to research is not actually that daunting. If drugs do arise that extend maximum lifespan, then the political will to classify aging as a disease might arise, in which case the FDA would have to classify aging as a disease and thus allow clinical trials of anti-aging drugs to proceed.

Other issues arise as well in this discussion, including the political and philosophical issues of anti-aging. Politically speaking, anti-aging medicine is complex. Issues

Department of Family and Community Medicine, Tulane University School of Medicine, 1430 Tulane Avenue TB-3, New Orleans, LA 70112, USA
E-mail address: atfort@tulane.edu

Clin Geriatr Med 27 (2011) 507–522
doi:10.1016/j.cger.2011.07.002
0749-0690/11/$ – see front matter © 2011 Elsevier Inc. All rights reserved.

of allotment of resources have the potential of overwhelming society. Already the entitlements promised to our older generations are demanding vast resources. These issues will continue to become more imminent as lifespan is prolonged. Perhaps someday we will have productive seven hundred year olds mentoring and providing resources for the sub-two century crowd, although before that time there are sure to be conflicts and perhaps even generational or economic warfare over resources to sustain vast populations who refuse to die.

Although this sounds like science fiction, some scientists embrace the possibility of millennial lifespans. If this were to happen, would it deprive new human life from the resources they require? Who will be entitled to the magical elixirs that may come forth in the study of biogerontology? Others argue that such a future is most unlikely and that there are finite limits to lifespan that will not be exceeded.

Where do you stand on these questions? What sort of moral issues might arise in a world populated with Methuselahs? Will the geriatric population enjoy a life of parasitic leisure provided by younger generations or will they provide for their own needs? Might it become true that the geriatric population enjoys such good health that they are the most productive members of society, while at the same time using the least resources? After all, they have wisdom and experience and are less likely to get bogged down in issues they learned to conquer years ago—issues that frustrate younger people, making them inefficient and unpredictable compared with more mature populations. Society may benefit in unimaginable ways from the influence and labors of the seasoned segment of the population. The traits of youth, although wonderful, are generally improved, having gone through the trials of experience.

All of these musings may be moot; it is currently true that despite all the optimism currently enjoyed by the anti-aging movement, it remains, at this time, according to the dictates of the scientific method, that there are no anti-aging medicines or any other processes that effectively extend maximum human lifespan.[1]

As physicians, we will be fielding many questions on these issues, so it behooves us to become familiar with biogerontology and the various ways it is represented. Which elements of this discipline enjoy legitimacy and which aspects are dubious? Although terms in this article are used almost interchangeably, there are some subtle contextual distinctions. The scientists and clinicians who remain in the domain of peer-reviewed research do not want to be associated with those proponents of anti-aging who profit off of dubious claims. Nor with those who twist research to manipulate consumers who are susceptible to their claims of providing actual extension of maximum human lifespan, as well as other too-good-to-be-true claims. The vast amount of quackery and financial fraud inflicted in the name of anti-aging is obviously not something one wishes to be associated with. We will try to further delineate these general distinctions at this time.

One school of thought holds that aging is a good and natural thing to be embraced as a necessary and positive aspect of life. To this school, aging, an inevitable process of decline, should be approached in a gentle, palliative way. This group trends toward improving the quality of existing lifespan and pursuing the idea of "compression of morbidity" (ie, minimalizing) time spent suffering from disease toward the end of a predominately healthy lifespan. This school of thought maintains standards in keeping with principles of the scientific method. These scientists study biogerontology and contribute to and may practice in the field of geriatrics. They aggressively research all aspects of aging with an open mind while remaining firmly grounded in the here and now. Although they are not opposed to science fiction, they are not investing in lots on the moon while they are still cheap. The material they produce is found in peer-reviewed, scientific journals and they remain unequivocally in the scientific milieu.

To others, aging is clearly a state of disease and should be vanquished or at least pushed as far into submission as human abilities are capable. Those who fall into this paradigm may generally be further split into 2 categories. One of these branches remains in the realm of legitimate hypothesis and proper scientific execution of ideas, whereas the other resides in the world of hyperbole.

Of these, the group that falls into the category of highly optimistic while remaining in the bounds of the accepted scientific arena, considers the human body to be a machine capable of restoration and repair, which could remain healthy for hundreds of years with proper maintenance and appropriate overhauls. A leader in this movement, Aubrey deGrey, PhD, a prominent biogerontologist at Oxford University, is quoted as follows: "Aging really is barbaric. It shouldn't be allowed. I don't need an ethical argument. I don't need any argument. It's visceral. To let people die is bad." He and other scientists have established the "Strategies for Engineered Negligible Senescence" (SENS foundation, which promotes the quest of rejuvenating the human body via an approach of tissue repair pursuant to the goal of a lifespan of a thousand years or more. This will be further elaborated in this article.

The other branch of the faction of those who wish to retard biological aging fall into a category of what is generally referred to as anti-aging medicine. These physicians and others who promote themselves as healers and scientists push regimens today that they claim will effectively extend lifespans. These regimens are often based on sophistry and frequently fool physicians as well as the lay public. Carefully selected scientific studies are often taken out of an appropriate frame of reference and distorted to construct an argument that safe and effective anti-aging remedies are currently available. Those who remain within the scientific purview argue that this third faction of anti-aging promoters siphon off resources and injure the reputation of biogerontology, thus impeding real progress in the field.

At any rate, this is a broad umbrella and covers a lot of territory; most certainly, it contains well-intentioned physicians as well as opportunistic hucksters. Many of these practitioners would certainly argue that they, too, are in the realm of legitimate applied science. Indeed many of their claims have been jumpstarted by scientific headlines, which are the basis of most of the hyperbole they trade in. For the most part, it seems that the current clinical practice of anti-aging medicine is built on a foundation of embellishment of scientific studies expanded out of context. Thus, real science is bound up with anti-aging claims, and to the lay public this seems to have a legitimate imprimatur of scientific authority.

A cursory look at internet offerings reveals a gamut—from shameless charlatanism combined with potentially dangerous hormones and drugs, to good preventative care practices mixed with some expensive supplements and laboratories that imply adherence with the principle of "primum non nocere." If one attends an anti-aging clinic that promotes healthy diet practices along with intelligent exercise, some expensive antioxidants, and a lot of personal attention, then one could perhaps argue this is good medicine, at least for the particular individual who might otherwise not be pursuing good health practices. However, it remains that the lay public who pursue anti-aging are entering a confusing realm with the difficult task of sorting out the wheat from the chaff. As a result, anti-aging medicine in general carries a stigmata, which is for the most part well deserved.

Nonetheless, as a clinician, questions about resveratrol, anti-oxidants, and other supplements will come your way. Queries on human growth hormone (HGH) and testosterone replacement will arise as patients are exposed to advertising by anti-aging institutes as well as pharmaceutical companies. Regardless of where one stands, the issue is huge and will be a prominent part of our lives. According to the

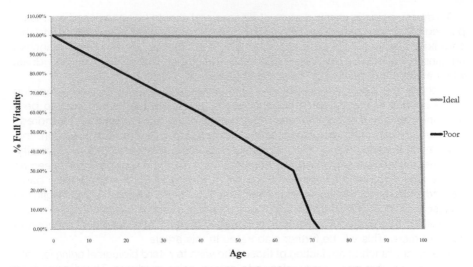

Fig. 1. Comparison of vitality between an ideal lifestyle and a poor lifestyle.

US census, the oldest old (ie, that segment of the population >85 years of age) is the fastest growing segment of our population. The elderly population in America is growing rapidly and will affect us all as we seek resources ourselves or contribute to providing resources for the care of our expanding geriatric population.

All of these approaches to lifespan should intersect at 1 point, namely, to extend the healthy proportion of one's lifespan to the maximum. This is often referred to as "compression of morbidity" or is also sometimes termed "rectangularization" of health and lifespan. Rectangularization portrays a line on a graph of vigorous health gradually declining over time grossly parallel with the horizontal line for age instead of a precipitous vertical decline in vitality in the range of middle age. Poor health causes the health line to plummet relative to the age line. This creates more of a triangular-ization of health and lifespan. Ideally, with good health, the health line runs almost parallel with the age line, thus approximating a rectangle. The idea is to compress the downward trend of health versus age as much as possible. The better one's health, the more parallel the lines of age and health will be (**Fig. 1**).

THEORIES OF AGING

What is aging? This depends on which theory of aging or combination thereof one subscribes to. The theory of cellular senescence proposes that cells finally lose the ability to divide simply by achieving the finite number of divisions they have been allotted.[2] These cell divisions are limited by the number of telomeres on the end of the cellular DNA. This is known as the Hayflick limit. There is a belief that this may present a good opportunity to intervene in the aging process. Might telomerase or some other strategy inhibit the loss of or even replace these telomeres and thus extend life? A current PubMed search for telomerase reveals 9861 research papers and the term telomere reveals 12,354 papers. This is clearly an area of interest.

Another theory is the free radical theory of aging, first proposed by Denham Harman in 1956. This theory proposes that cumulative damage from free radicals finally overcomes a cell's ability to repair itself, leading to cell death and eventually to the death of the organism.[3] Free radicals are a byproduct of the normal metabolism of living as well as a byproduct of environmental insults such as radiation, toxic exposures, and dietary indiscretions. The public consciousness is well ingrained with the idea that antioxidants are good for delaying aging. Antioxidants offer themselves sacrificially so that they are oxidized instead of our body's cells. The free radical theory of aging continues to be revised by Harman and others, and remains a strong theory. The more free radicals are studied, the more complex the related questions become. Recent thinking makes the consumption of antioxidants uncertain. It seems that taking antioxidants might not be a healthy thing to do after all. A certain level of free radical activity might be necessary to carry out restorative and physiologic functions in the body.[4] Thus, the answer to the antioxidant supplementation question is not clear, although free radicals are without doubt a part of the riddle of aging. For more on this subject, see the articles on toxins, diet, and vitamins and supplements.

Another compelling idea is the "glycation theory of aging," which has been described as a caramelization of tissues. This theory purports that "advanced glycation endproducts" (AGEs), a sugar and protein matrix much augmented by chronic hyperglycemia, essentially gums up the works.[5] These AGEs are thought to cross-link proteins, causing them to become ineffective in their various purposes, which leads to wrinkles, inflammation, cataracts, and other undesirable processes. This theory seems to be consistent with our modern, high-carbohydrate lifestyle and is even more pronounced among diabetics, who have more sugar available for glycation.[6] As a corollary, it is thought that calorie restriction (CR), proven to extend lifespan in animals, works in part by decreasing AGEs resulting in improved cell maintenance and increased longevity.

Another theory promotes the primacy of mitochondrial decay in aging.[7] Mitochondrial damage occurs secondary to everything from the accumulation of destruction by free radicals and the resultant genetic errors, to the toxic accumulation of metabolic waste byproducts. At some point, the mitochondria are no longer able to provide energy to the organism from oxidative metabolism, and even contribute further to the organism's decay via their own breakdown as they emit waste and free radicals. When these symbiotic organelles are no longer able to withstand the oxidative stress of metabolism, aging rapidly ensues.

It seems reasonable to infer that the accumulation of errors from all of the above theories, adds up to increased cell damage, overall entropy, and eventual aging. These theories of aging form the basis for ideas to increase lifespan, as well as decrease morbidity in advanced age.

Before advancing into stratagems for life extension and compression of morbidity, it is notable that we already have a vast and capable anti-aging network established. This consists of public health practices, vaccines, and primary care medicine. The average lifespan in Western countries was increased by 30 years during the 20th century owing to public health practices.[8] If one consistently complies with public health paradigms, one can already expect a relatively long life. Medicines such as anti-hypertensives, blood sugar modulators, and lipid modifiers certainly qualify as cutting-edge anti-aging medicines for those who require them, because they suppress diseases known to shorten lifespan. They also often amount to the same thing people are seeking in futuristic anti-aging medicines, a way to circumvent aging and disease without bothering to change one's lifestyle. This seems to be the American way or, should I say, human way, and probably drives much of the purported annual $50 billion spent on anti-aging medicine at this time. At this point, those pursuing the easy way to longevity (ie, not putting in the time or effort) will probably reap little in the way of quality longevity. That being said, let's delve into what is being offered.

CALORIE RESTRICTION

CR is 1 life extension strategy that consistently stands up against the scientific method. Numerous studies confirm that "calorie restriction with adequate nutrition" is indeed, proven to lengthen mammalian lifespans.[9,10] This is obviously a promising avenue for exploration in humans. CR increases lifespan in lower life forms, as well as dogs and rodents, and is being extensively studied in non-human primates.[11,12] The obvious hope is that its effects will apply to humans as well. Human studies are ongoing at this time.[13]

CR first came to light in 1934 when rats, fed a low-calorie diet with adequate nutrition, lived as much as twice as long as rats on a conventional diet. Multiple experiments have ascertained that CR proportionally increases quantity and quality of life in rats and mice.[9,10] The positive effects of CR are myriad and have been documented extensively. For example, the risk of atherosclerotic disease is clearly diminished.[14] Body mass index, of course, decreases. Memory improves in the elderly.[15] In 1 study, blood pressure markedly decreased to about 100/60 in the CR group, and low-density lipoprotein and total cholesterol decreased below all but the bottom 10% of the population. The average high-density lipoprotein was in the top 85th to 90th percentile for middle-aged American men.[14] Along with this, a decrease in body temperature was noted. Fasting plasma insulin and glucose levels dropped off significantly along with inflammatory markers such as C-reactive protein.[14] These are just some of the benefits. CR, at this time, seems to hold great promise in the field of anti-aging.

In addition to these effects on individual parameters, CR is also thought to have "system-wide effects." Because CR lowers metabolic activity,[16] it is, in effect, slowing down the "mechanism of living," thereby reducing oxidative stress and slowing cellular division. In addition, the slight amount of oxidative stress actually brought on by CR is thought to "prime" the individual and make it more ready it to fight off more harmful sources of oxidation. In other words, a little defensive stress keeps the organism functioning optimally. This is also known as hormesis.

Additionally, CR activates the silent information receptor 2 (SIR2) and SIRT1 through SIRT7 (mammalian versions are SIRT) genes producing proteins known as sirtuins, which are proposed to advance anti-aging effects.[17] Sirtuins are thought to work by silencing certain genes in response to stress, especially the stress of CR. Thus, the sirtuins are thought by some to be the key to the benefits of CR.

Resveratrol

This leads to the obvious question of how to exploit the possibilities offered by CR. One promising offering on the horizon are the CR mimetic drugs. These are natural and pharmaceutical attempts to mimic CR diets. In other words, one may enjoy the benefits of CR while still eating as one wishes. Resveratrol has been the most studied candidate for anti-aging via mimicking CR and is believed to work via activation of sirtuin-producing genes. Resveratrol is produced in grapevines and some other plants as a defensive reaction to a stressful environment. It is hypothesized that these defensive properties may be exploited for use in humans as well. Red wine, as well as a plant called knotweed, contains a relatively large amount of resveratrol. Resveratrol first gained attention as a possible explanation of the "French paradox," explaining the French population's health and vitality despite the regular consumption of wine and foods considered by some in the United States to be incongruous with optimum health practices. Resveratrol is extensively studied; a PubMed search shows that it is a constituent of 3751 research papers. Its benefits are controversial and by no means clear,[18,19] and yet it remains among the most studied avenues in the school of CR mimetics. Resveratrol has been shown to increase lifespan in lower life forms as well as in obese mice,[20-22] although there is currently no conclusive evidence that it will extend lifespan in humans.

Aside from activating sirtuin-producing genes, resveratrol seems to have other beneficial effects such as antioxidant,[23] antiviral,[24] anticarcinogenic,[25] antidiabetic,[26] and anti-inflammatory effects,[27] as well as cardioprotective[28] and neuroprotective effects.[29] The accumulation of all these positive effects would seem to almost certainly lead to compression of morbidity, as well as potentially lending credence to life extension with resveratrol via other mechanisms than sirtuin activation alone. Paradoxically, there is some research indicating that it may be carcinogenic as well.[30] Currently, resveratrol remains highly studied as a potential venue to promote good health and longevity.

It is of note that the pharmaceutical company, Sirtris, a branch of GlaxoSmithKline, halted clinical trials of resveratrol in December 2010. Resveratrol itself is not patentable; an article in *The New York Times* stated that this is 1 reason for the halt, as well as the idea that the company will now concentrate on SIRT1 and patentable activators of SIRT, which have resulted from the study of resveratrol.[31] The doses of resveratrol that produced results in mice are comparable with the amount a human would consume by drinking 300 glasses of wine per day. There must be a better way, and Sirtris believes it is via sirtuin activators. These activators, it is hoped, will mimic the famine reflex in organisms, which is believed to be the underlying source of the life extension effects of CR.

Rapamycin

Another promising CR mimetic candidate is rapamycin, an immunosuppressant shown to extend life in invertebrates and mice.[32] Rapamycin is named for Easter island (*Rapa Nui*), where it was found in soil samples in the streptomyces family of bacteria. Rapamycin is currently used as an immunosuppresant inhibiting transplant rejection. Although it seems to have great promise, it may be that these immune system–inhibiting properties would be difficult to overcome if it were proven useful as an anti-aging medicine. Most importantly, it elucidated the target of rapamycin (TOR) gene's role in aging.

It is thought that rapamycin may prevent aging in basically the same ways as CR does. Rapamycin inhibits the TOR gene(s), which seems to have a broad role in anti-aging/CR–type effects. TOR seems to control aspects of protein production and, as such, ceases production of proteins under times of stress. TOR is akin to an on/off switch for a cascade of cellular mechanisms that, it turns out, are consistent with what happens in CR. This, in turn, is thought to be a life-extending process. TOR genes, when inhibited, as with rapamycin or CR, cause a chain of complex and varied life-extending stress responses.[33]

Rapamycin and resveratrol show promise as CR mimetics, although they are far from being proven to extend lifespan or improve quality of life in humans. For now, they remain in the realm of research and great potential. They may be most significant in that they catalyzed discovery of cellular gene expressions, which are activated by indicators of stress, and when activated facilitate life-extending response to these stressors. These gene targets are just the surface and may be able to be exploited in other ways in the future. This being said, resveratrol currently enjoys widespread consumption and enthusiastic proponents and continues to receive generous research funding.

Metformin

Metformin is a CR mimetic in many ways. One study promotes it as a life extender via tumor inhibition.[34] Predominately, it functions in life extension as a blood glucose-lowering agent. In accordance with current knowledge, metformin only promotes life extension by suppressing the lifespan-shortening disease processes of diabetes, although it may turn out to be a maximum life extension drug as well. Metformin works in multiple ways to disrupt the effects of high calorie consumption as well as cause beneficial genetic expression of proteins to occur. Metformin is known to both increase the number of insulin receptors, as well as upgrade the performance of insulin receptors. It inhibits absorption of glucose by the gut and at the same time inhibits gluconeogenesis, both serving to lower blood glucose and the myriad negative effects of hyperglycemia. Metformin reduces gene expression of enzymes that increase oxidation of fatty acids, which, in turn, leads to retarding cellular death.[35] It also activates gene expression of proteins, which regulate glycolysis in a beneficial manner. All of these processes are beneficial to avoid glycation and thus AGEs. Finally, metformin activates adenosine monophosphate-activated protein kinase (AMP-K), an enzyme participating in cellular repair. This enzyme, which is also activated by other processes such as CR, has a direct CR mimetic function.[36] Even if all of these discoveries were not available, it might be said that, secondary to the gluttonous dietary practices in play today, metformin belongs as a potential candidate in the anti-aging pantheon.

There are other substances that might be added to the CR mimetic pipeline, but none currently promising enough or adequately peer reviewed to elicit mention in this overview.

EXERCISE

Another avenue for exploration is exercise. Exercise is or should be a major player in an anti-aging or compression of morbidity program. Please refer to the article on exercise for a more in-depth analysis. The effects of exercise are unquestionably beneficial as long as pursued in a reasonable manner. To begin with, exercise has some of the same properties as CR, such as increasing insulin receptor sensitivity,[37] lowering blood glucose levels,[38] and blood lipid levels.[39] Exercise increases muscle mass and strength,[40] builds bone density,[41,42] and lowers blood pressure[43] in addition to increasing a sense of well-being.[44] Exercise also lowers cortisol levels,[45] which in turn reduces the negative effects of hypersecretion of cortisol, the "stress hormone."

Excess cortisol can result in the metabolic syndrome, decreased bone density, insomnia, and depression, all of which serve to impede good health.[46] Vigorous exercise also releases both testosterone and HGH, as well as beneficial physiologic cortisol.[47] Regular exercise has clear benefits. Exercise releases the stress enzyme AMP-K, as previously.[48] Regular exercise maintains increased insulin receptor sensitivity, which then lowers plasma insulin levels and potentiates all of the benefits that follow from lowering insulin levels. A discussion of exercise and its relation to insulin presents a good opportunity to discuss the negative effects of elevated insulin levels as a result of insulin insensitivity. Insulin:

- Increases production of triglycerides.
- Forces fat tissues to make and store fat.
- Decreases the breakdown of fats for energy metabolism.
- Decreases gluconeogenesis, which utilizes energy stores in the liver.
- Decreases autophagy and, thus, destruction of damaged organelles.

Conversely, when insulin is not available, fat is metabolized as an energy source. Although exercise has not been shown to extend life in an absolute way, it is clear that by association with its myriad effects that multiple benefits are accrued from exercise. It has many positive physiologic effects that promote characteristics consistent with longer and healthier lives. Once again, as with our primary care medicines, exercise may be said to extend individual life in the sense that it inhibits diseases that are known to shorten life.

THE SENS STRATEGY

One of the more compelling arguers for anti-aging is Aubrey de Grey, PhD, the founder of the SENS Foundation. He publishes the academic journal *Rejuvenation Research*, a peer-reviewed journal that can be found through PubMed. He has also authored *The Mitochondrial Free Radical Theory of Aging* and co-authored *Endless Aging*. The basis of all his efforts is the SENS strategy—"Strategies for Engineered Negligible Senescence"—a plan to repair or rejuvenate what he considers to be the 7 causes of senescence. Dr de Grey believes that if his plan can be implemented, then we may enjoy healthy lifespans of perhaps thousands of years. He believes science to be on the threshold of this if society will put the resources and effort into it. Although many have attempted to portray his ideas as untenable, his theories withstand criticism and no one has been able to box him outside of the scientific arena.[49] The MIT Technology Review magazine offered a significant monetary prize in 2006 for anyone who could effectively debunk his proposals. No one has yet collected the money.[50]

The SENS strategy has a 7-point plan to address what Dr de Grey considers the 7 biological processes leading to the entropy of aging, paraphrased as follows:

- Tissue degeneration occurs as a result of advancing age. This is especially important in vital organs such as the heart and brain. Regenerative medicine and stem cell research are currently addressing this issue.
- Telomere-related mechanisms leading to cancer through immortalization of cancer cells must be selectively modified using targeted gene therapies. Dr de Grey proposes modifying telomere modification genes according to tissue type. This would enable us to deactivate the immortality mechanism of cancer cells, thereby curing the cancer.
- Mitochondrial DNA lies outside the cellular nucleus and this extranuclear exposure leads to accumulated damage. Dr de Grey proposes copying mitochondrial DNA into the cellular nucleus via gene therapy in an effort to maintain its functions in an optimal manner. Other strategies to the same effect are also being pursued.
- Certain proteins in our bodies are very long lived. At the same time that they persist in our bodies, they also become ineffective junk or poor-quality substrates for whatever function they should or did perform. Science should seek out catalysts to eliminate fatigued elements while inducing their replacements.
- Senescent cells of certain types often accumulate in unwanted areas, such as joint spaces, impeding optimum mechanical or physiologic functions, which lead to symptoms of degenerative aging. Creating immune responses via our own immune cells to eliminate these cells would alleviate this problem.
- In a similar vein, junk material known as amyloid accumulates outside of our cells in our interstitium (eg, amyloid is evident in Alzheimer's patients). Other sorts of extracellular junk also accumulate. Vaccines to incite active immunity against this "junk" are currently being researched.

- Some human cells are very long-lived and non-dividing; yet another sort of junk accumulates in these cells serving to foul up optimal functioning. Dr de Grey proposes a search for nontoxic, microbial enzymes in soil bacteria to be introduced into aging cells to eliminate these wastes, thus restoring optimal function.

"Junk" as the term is used in this theory is actually very specific and contextual; the nomenclature is a convenient tool. The different sorts of junk require differing solutions. The technology to implement the above strategy is either extant or nascent and is not all that far-fetched as per Dr de Grey.

The SENS strategy does not fall into the mainstream biogerontology academy or the snake oil academy. de Grey et al are in a realm of their own making and clearly not to be ignored. Dr de Grey notes that our knowledge base is currently beginning to expand exponentially which can only be auspicious for futuristic endeavors. Stay tuned.

CLINICS AND THERAPIES

Anti-aging clinics, of varying degrees of quality and intent, are available and easily accessed today for those who are interested. There is no easy way to establish a clear line between greedy opportunism and well-meaning sincerity without personal experience, extensive study, or perhaps word of mouth. Most clinics do not openly reveal their regimens. A thorough study of the peer-reviewed literature should be undertaken by anyone before participating in anti-aging medicine modalities at this time. Well-meaning practitioners may be pushing worthless elixirs, whereas others may be selling regimens that they promote with firm conviction regardless of any effects, positive or negative. Various clinics offer differing solutions to aging. Most seem, from a cursory Internet investigation, to involve HGH and other hormone assays and possible treatments, along with various supplements, perhaps accompanied by lifestyle changes. A thorough exploration of these clinics and what occurs in the name of anti-aging is in order.

HGH

On the 1 hand, the promise of resveratrol is tempting and in small doses seems to have little downside; on the other hand, HGH became all the rage after 1 study[51] and remains controversial. HGH is said to foment muscle growth, cellular reproduction, and regeneration in humans and is now available via recombinant DNA technology. It has been used by athletes to augment performance and is tested for in the Olympics and other sporting venues for its anabolic effects. A study in the New England Journal of Medicine in 1990 initiated HGH into the anti-aging pantheon. The 12 men greater than 60 years old who took HGH developed markedly increased muscle mass and bone density; the control group showed no improvement.[51] Regardless of these findings, the author in no way claimed that it was an anti-aging drug and even argued against that premise. A later study at Stanford University showed an increase in muscle mass with an equivalent decrease in fat tissue, but no increase in strength. No other positive indicators of improved fitness were noted.[52] It is important to note that HGH may increase the risk of diabetes, and contribute to arthralgia, edema, carpal tunnel syndrome, and gynecomastia.[52] The FDA only approves its use for growth hormone deficiency in adults or children. The loophole around this is that HGH deficiency may be diagnosed on symptoms alone; thus, it is not necessarily based on an objective measurement. The bottom line on HGH is caveat emptor. As long as the anti-aging patient is aware of the tenuousness and possibly negative aspects of treatment, then the decision should become reasonable for the individual and his or her physician. Please refer to the article on hormone replacement for more on this subject.

Testosterone

Testosterone has also been a part of the anti-aging repertoire since the publication of Paul deKruif's "The Male Hormone" in 1945.[53] The term andropause is a popular way to attribute some aging characteristics to the decrease in testosterone that occurs normally with aging. Among testosterone's benefits, it is known to increase muscle mass and strength, increase bone density and strength, as well as decrease the risk of type 2 diabetes, obesity, depression, cardiovascular disease, and possibly Alzheimer's disease.[54] Testosterone is said to increase energy, libido, erythropoiesis, and general well-being. Testosterone is an anabolic steroid, which imparts physiologic and psychological advantages in sports and other arenas.[55–57]

Obviously, testosterone is very appealing and many consider it to be safe. The truth is that it is not yet clear if replacing testosterone for andropause is a completely benign endeavor.[58] One commonly believed downside of supplementation is the risk of prostate cancer. However, there is evidence that prostate cancer risk is no higher in men with low testosterone levels,[59] who are given supplementation. Further data trend toward the idea that there is no relationship between high testosterone levels and prostate cancer risk.[60] At the same time, it cannot be said with unequivocal certainty that testosterone does not increase any form of cancer risk. The exposure to hormone replacement in men is nowhere near that experienced with hormone replacement therapy in women. The sheer volume of exposure is not there, and it took a long time and a lot of exposure years in women to become fully aware of the dangers involved.

Furthermore, testosterone has noted benefits for women, including treating sexual dysfunction, dysmenorrhea, and abnormal uterine bleeding, as well as possible anti-tumoral activity. Testosterone has been used for decades in all of these roles.[61] Conversely, there is currently evidence that exogenous testosterone may have serious side effects in women,[62] although for the most part if used judiciously, it has been considered safe.[63,64] On the other hand, women have been given estrogen replacement therapy for decades, and although harmful effects have now been proved, it still is an individual decision as to whether or not the risk benefit ratio is acceptable. Similarly, with testosterone, the answer is again caveat emptor. A well-informed patient, armed with a recent and thorough review article, should make a reasonable decision regarding the risks and benefits of testosterone and proceed from there.

Dehydroepiandrosterone

Dehydroepiandrosterone (DHEA) is secreted by the adrenal glands, gonads, and brain. It is a steroid hormone that acts directly and via its metabolites to stimulate androgen receptors. DHEA is said to be a precursor of the sex steroids and many benefits are purported to accrue from its use.

The *Journal of the American Geriatrics Society* in June 2008 published a study in which researchers conclude that lower levels of DHEA-s correlate with a shorter lifespan, and higher levels of DHEA-s are a strong predictor of longevity in men.[65] The obvious opportunistic extrapolation evident from this is that it may be interpreted that higher levels might extend lifespan.

A study in the *New England Journal of Medicine* in 2006 states that, "Neither DHEA nor low-dose testosterone replacement in elderly people has physiologically relevant beneficial effects on body composition, physical performance, insulin sensitivity, or quality of life."[66] DHEA is the adrenal gland's main steroid secretion and may be metabolized to estrogen or testosterone in the body. Its use as a supplement is illegal in the Olympics and other venues, and requires a prescription in Canada. Its unrestricted use is protected in the United States because it is classified as a dietary supplement and thus free of FDA approval before use.[67]

Many claims are made on behalf of DHEA. It is said to be a cortisol antagonist and a depression fighter.[68] Some claim it is a performance enhancer, although there is no evidence of this. It is said to be a cancer agonist,[69] as well as a cancer antagonist.[70] It is also said to be advantageous in cardiovascular disease[71] and possibly helpful in type 2 diabetics with atherosclerotic disease.[72]

The negative effects of DHEA mirror those of testosterone replacement. It is a complex compound and not completely understood. DHEA may have negative qualities, while at the same time showing very little evidence of any positive qualities when used outside of the scope of its normal human physiologic function. A recent review study found no benefits in anti-aging from the use of DHEA.[64] This is another example of a supplement that should be warily approached and individually decided upon.

SUMMARY

It has been said that if cancer were eradicated this would extend our modern Western lifespans by about 3 years.[73] The consensus of many leaders in aging science today is that an extension of the average maximum lifespan to 100 years, via anti-aging medicine, if possible is a long way off, and will not be available to anyone alive today.[74] Despite this, our culture is very much invested with a love of science fiction. We all know of culturally inculcated tales of how wrong the scientific establishment has often been. Most of us are aware of the persecution of Galileo for opposing the geocentric view of the universe. We hear examples of the detractors who thought it preposterous we could land on the moon given to us as lessons for life in childhood and beyond. Physicians resisted Lister's antiseptic technique until its truth was unavoidable. Imposing these historical examples of reactionary science on the anti-aging dialectic may just be more hyperbole. Yet, whether or not these examples are currently relevant to anti-aging medicine, one can be assured this thought paradigm will remain relevant to modern psyches. We will remain suspicious of those who doubt the future glories of science. Science is a considerable icon in our society, and one in which most of us have invested vast faith. Futuristic science is a proud part of our cultural identity. Because of this, it is virtually guaranteed that many will continue to pursue and promote anti-aging research and medicine in all her guises, both reasoned and otherwise. Considering this, it seems evident that biogerontology's many forms will continue to proliferate and, like most things, it is unpredictable where they may lead.

In conclusion, as a responsible physician one is compelled to acquire a reasonably broad understanding of what is occurring in the wide world of anti-aging now and feasibly in the future. An interesting exercise is an Internet search for anti-aging, which opens a kaleidoscope of compilations of varying quality and purpose. Typing in the word "anti-aging" almost instantly retrieves 19 million citations on Google. One needs to be well-informed to sort through all of this.

What is apparent from the scientific research available today is that there are positive medical practices and lifestyle choices that can extend our individual lives. The caveat here is that they only do so at present by inhibiting processes that shorten our individual lifespans. There is no evidence that any of what is currently available actually extends our maximum potential lifespan. The best current idea might be that by living the best possible disease-inhibiting lifestyle, some among us may make 120 years of age. This is predicated on supercentenarian Jeanne Calment's 122-year lifespan.[75]

As a general rule, the best possible outcome a physician can offer his patients is compression of morbidity and inhibition of age-accelerating disease to extend individual lives quantitatively and qualitatively. As a result of a study of this text, it is hoped that the reader is ready and prepared to navigate all of the offerings thrust at us in this time where the fastest growing demographic are the oldest old. The first baby boomers reached age 65 in 2011, and it is safe to predict this group will be pursuing the subject of life extension. We wish our readers good luck as they endeavor to lead others through the process of aging gracefully and well. We hope this text helps our readers to effectively develop a reasoned and well-informed opinion while still retaining an open mind. With all the resources and interest in extending lifespan there is no doubt much more to come.

REFERENCES

1. Butler RN, Fossel M, Harman SM, et al. Is there an anti-aging medicine? J Gerontol A Biol Sci Med Sci 2002;57:B333–8.
2. Jiang H, Ju Z, Rudolph KL. Telomere shortening and ageing. Z Gerontol Geriatr 2007;40:314–24.
3. Harman D. Aging: a theory based on free radical and radiation chemistry. J Gerontol 1956;11:298–300.
4. Bjelakovic G, Nikolova D, Gluud LL, et al. Antioxidant supplements for prevention of mortality in healthy participants and patients with various diseases. Cochrane Database Syst Rev 2008;2:CD007176.
5. Meerwaldt R, Links T, Zeebregts C, et al. The clinical relevance of assessing advanced glycation endproducts accumulation in diabetes. Cardiovasc Diabetol 2008;7:29.
6. Vlassara H. Advanced glycation in health and disease: role of the modern environment. Ann N Y Acad Sci 2005;1043:452–60.
7. Romano AD, Serviddio G, de Matthaeis A, et al. Oxidative stress and aging. J Nephrol 2010;23(Suppl 15):S29–36.
8. Control and prevention. Ten great public health achievements—United States, 1900–1999. JAMA 1999;281:1481.
9. McCay CM, Crowell MF. Prolonging the life span. The Scientific Monthly 1934;39:405–14.
10. Bordone L, Guarente L. Calorie restriction, SIRT1 and metabolism: understanding longevity. Nat Rev Mol Cell Biol 2005;6:298–305.
11. Mair W, Goymer P, Pletcher SD, et al. Demography of dietary restriction and death in Drosophila. Science 2003;301:1731–3.
12. Colman RJ, Beasley TM, Allison DB, et al. Attenuation of sarcopenia by dietary restriction in rhesus monkeys. J Gerontol A Biol Sci Med Sci 2008;63:556–9.
13. Rochon J, Bales CW, Ravussin E, et al. Design and conduct of the CALERIE study: comprehensive assessment of the long-term effects of reducing intake of energy. J Gerontol A Biol Sci Med Sci. 2011;66:97–108.
14. Fontana L, Meyer TE, Klein S, et al. Long term calorie restriction is highly effective in reducing the risk for atherosclerosis in humans. Proc Natl Acad Sci U S A 2004;101:6659–63.
15. Witte AV, Fobker M, Gellner R, et al. Caloric restriction improves memory in elderly humans. Proc Natl Acad Sci U S A 2009;106:1255–60.

16. Roth GS, Ingram DK, Lane MA. Calorie restriction in primates and relevance to humans. Ann N Y Acad Sci 2001;928:305–15.
17. Satoh A, Brace CS, Ben-Josef G, et al. SIRT1 promotes the central adaptive response to diet restriction through activation of the dorsomedial and lateral nuclei of the hypothalamus. J Neurosci 2010;30:10220–32.
18. Fremont L. Biological effects of resveratrol. Life Sci 2000;66:663–73.
19. Mukherjee S, Dudley JI, Das DK. Dose dependency of resveratrol in providing health benefits. Dose Response 2010;8:478–500.
20. Howitz KT, Bitterman KJ, Cohen HY, et al. Small molecule activators of sirtuins extend Saccharomyces cerevisiae lifespan. Nature 2003;425:191–6.
21. Wood JG, Rogina B, Lavu S, et al. Sirtuin activators mimic caloric restriction and delay ageing in metazoans. Nature 2004;430:686–9.
22. Valenzano DR, Terzibasi E, Genade T, et al. Resveratrol prolongs lifespan and retards the onset of age-related markers in a short-lived vertebrate. Curr Biol 2006;16:296–300.
23. Hung LM, Chen JK, Huang SS, et al. Cardioprotective effect of resveratrol, a natural antioxidant derived from grapes. Cardiovasc Res 2000;47:549–55.
24. Docherty JJ, Sweet TJ, Bailey E, et al. Resveratrol inhibition of varicella-zoster virus replication in vitro. Antiviral Res 2006;72:171–7.
25. Leone S, Cornetta T, Basso E, et al. Resveratrol induces DNA double-strand breaks through human topoisomerase II interaction. Cancer Lett 2010;295:167–72.
26. Deng JY, Hsieh PS, Huang JP, et al. Activation of estrogen receptor is crucial for resveratrol-stimulating muscular glucose uptake via both insulin-dependent and -independent pathways. Diabetes 2008;57:1814–23.
27. Gentilli M, Mazoit JX, Bouaziz H, et al. Resveratrol decreases hyperalgesia induced by carrageenan in the rat hind paw. Life Sci 2001;68:1317–21.
28. Kopp P. Resveratrol, a phytoestrogen found in red wine. A possible explanation for the conundrum of the 'French paradox'? Eur J Endocrinol 1998;138:619–20.
29. Karuppagounder SS, Pinto JT, Xu H, et al. Dietary supplementation with resveratrol reduces plaque pathology in a transgenic model of Alzheimer's disease. Neurochem Int 2009;54:111–8.
30. Gehm BD, McAndrews JM, Chien PY, et al. Resveratrol, a polyphenolic compound found in grapes and wine, is an agonist for the estrogen receptor. Proc Natl Acad Sci U S A 1997;94:14138–43.
31. Wade N. Doubt on anti-aging molecule as drug trial stops. The New York Times Science, January 10, 2011.
32. Harrison DE, Strong R, Sharp ZD, et al. Rapamycin fed late in life extends lifespan in genetically heterogeneous mice. Nature 2009;460:392–5.
33. Stanfel MN, Shamieh LS, Kaeberlein M, et al. The TOR pathway comes of age. Biochim Biophys Acta 2009;1790:1067–74.
34. Anisimov VN, Berstein LM, Egormin PA, et al. Effect of metformin on life span and on the development of spontaneous mammary tumors in HER-2/neu transgenic mice. Exp Gerontol 2005;40:685–93.
35. Collier CA, Bruce CR, Smith AC, et al. Metformin counters the insulin-induced suppression of fatty acid oxidation and stimulation of triacylglycerol storage in rodent skeletal muscle. Am J Physiol Endocrinol Metab 2006;291:E182–9.
36. Gaochao Z, Myers R, Li Y, et al. Role of AMP-activated protein kinase in mechanism of metformin action. J Clin Invest 2001;108:1167–74.
37. Borghouts LB, Keizer HA. Exercise and insulin sensitivity: a review. Int J Sports Med 2000;21:1–12.

38. Sigal RJ, Kenny GP, Boulé NG, et al. Effects of aerobic training, resistance training, or both on glycemic control in type 2 diabetes: a randomized trial. Ann Intern Med 2007;147:357–69.
39. Kelly RB. Diet and exercise in the management of hyperlipidemia. Am Fam Physician 2010;81:1097–102.
40. Phillips SM. Physiologic and molecular bases of muscle hypertrophy and atrophy: impact of resistance exercise on human skeletal muscle (protein and exercise dose effects). Appl Physiol Nutr Metab 2009;34:403–10.
41. American College of Sports Medicine position stand. Osteoporosis and exercise. Med Sci Sports Exerc 1995;27:i–vii.
42. Zehnacker CH, Bemis-Dougherty A. Effect of weighted exercises on bone mineral density in post menopausal women. A systematic review. J Geriatr Phys Ther 2007;30:79–88.
43. Fagard RH. Exercise is good for your blood pressure: effects of endurance training and resistance training. Clin Exp Pharmacol Physiol 2006;33:853–6.
44. Hassmen P, Kolvula N, Uutela A. Physical exercise and psychological well-being. A study in Finland. Prev Med 2000;30:17–25.
45. Wellhoener P, Born J, Fehm H, et al. Elevated resting and exercise induced cortisol levels after mineralocorticoid receptor blockade with canrenoate in healthy humans. J Clin Endocrinol Metab 2004;89:5048–52.
46. Reini SA. Hypercortisolism as a potential concern for submariners. Aviat Space Environ Med 2010;81:1114–22.
47. Smilios I, Pilianidis T, Karamouzis M, et al. Hormonal responses after a strength endurance resistance exercise protocol in young and elderly males. Int J Sports Med 2007;28:401–6.
48. Winder WW, Hardie DG. AMP-activated protein kinase, a metabolic master switch: possible roles in type 2 diabetes. Am J Physiol 1999;277:E1–10.
49. Nuland S. Do you want to live forever. MIT Technology Review. Feb 2005.
50. Pontin J. Is defeating aging only a dream? MIT Technology Review. July 11, 2006.
51. Rudman D, Feller AG, Nagraj HS, et al. Effects of human growth hormone in men over 60 years old. N Engl J Med 1990;323:1–6.
52. Liu H, Bravata DM, Olkin I, et al. Systematic review: the safety and efficacy of growth hormone in the healthy elderly. Ann Intern Med 2007;146:104–15.
53. de Kruif P. The Male Hormone. New York: Harcourt, Brace; 1945.
54. Rosario ER, Carroll J, Pike CJ. Testosterone regulation of Alzheimer-like neuropathology in male 3xTg-AD mice involves both estrogen and androgen pathways. Brain Res 2010;1359:281–90.
55. Bassil N, Morley JE. Late-life onset hypogonadism: a review. Clin Geriatr Med 2010;26:197–222.
56. Zitzmann M. Testosterone deficiency, insulin resistance and the metabolic syndrome. Nat Rev Endocrinol 2009;5:673–81.
57. Saad F. The role of testosterone in type 2 diabetes and metabolic syndrome in men. Arq Bras Endocrinol Metab 2009;53:901–7.
58. Calof OM, Singh AB, Lee ML, et al. Adverse events associated with testosterone replacement in middle-aged and older men: a meta-analysis of randomized, placebo-controlled trials. J Gerontol A Biol Sci Med Sci 2005;60:1451–7.
59. Morgentaler A. Testosterone replacement therapy and prostate risks: where's the beef? Can J Urol 2006;13(Suppl 1):40–3.
60. Raynaud JP. Prostate cancer risk in testosterone-treated men. J Steroid Biochem Mol Biol 2006;102:261–6.

61. Traish AM, Feeley RJ, Guay AT. Testosterone therapy in women with gynecological and sexual disorders: a triumph of clinical endocrinology from 1938 to 2008. J Sex Med 2009;6:334–51.
62. Dizon DS, Tejada-Berges T, Koelliker S, et al. Ovarian cancer associated with testosterone supplementation in a female-to-male transsexual patient. Gynecol Obstet Invest 2006;62:226–8.
63. Bolour S, Braunstein G. Testosterone therapy in women: a review. Int J Impot Res 2005;17:399–408.
64. Kritz-Silverstein D, von Mühlen D, Laughlin GA, et al. Effects of dehydroepiandrosterone supplementation on cognitive function and quality of life: the DHEA and Well-Ness (DAWN) Trial. J Am Geriatr Soc 2008;56:1292–8.
65. Enomoto M, Adachi H, Fukami A, et al. Serum dehydroepiandrosterone sulfate levels predict longevity in men: 27-year follow-up study in a community-based cohort (Tanushimaru study). J Am Geriatr Soc 2008;56:994–8.
66. Nair KS, Rizza RA, O'Brien P, et al. DHEA in Elderly Women and DHEA or Testosterone in Elderly Men. N Engl J Med 2006;355:1647–59.
67. Goldman P. Herbal medicines today and the roots of modern pharmacology. Ann Intern Med 2001;135:594–600.
68. Gallagher P, Young A. Cortisol/DHEA ratios in depression. Neuropsychopharmacology 2002;26:410.
69. Key T, Appleby P, Barnes I, et al. Endogenous sex hormones and breast cancer in postmenopausal women: reanalysis of nine prospective studies. J Natl Cancer Inst 2002;94:606–16.
70. Schulz S, Klann RC, Schönfeld S, et al. Mechanisms of cell growth inhibition and cell cycle arrest in human colonic adenocarcinoma cells by dehydroepiandrosterone: role of isoprenoid biosynthesis. Cancer Res 1992;52:1372–6.
71. Barrett-Connor E, Khaw KT, Yen SS. A prospective study of dehydroepiandrosterone sulfate, mortality, and cardiovascular disease. N Engl J Med 1986;315:1519–24.
72. Fukui M, Kitagawa Y, Nakamura N, et al. Serum dehydroepiandrosterone and sulfate concentration and carotid atherosclerosis in men with type 2 diabetes. Atherosclerosis 2005;181:339–44.
73. Yashin AI, Ukraintseva SV, Akushevich IV, et al. Trade-off between cancer and aging: what role do other diseases play? Evidence from experimental and human population studies. Mech Ageing Dev 2009;130:98–104.
74. Olshansky SJ, Carnes BA, Désesquelles A. Demography. Prospects for human longevity. Science 2001;291:1491–2.
75. Coles LS. Demography of human supercentenarians. J Gerontol A Biol Sci Med Sci 2004;59:B579–86.

Aging and Disease Prevention

Roger J. Zoorob, MD, MPH[a],*, Courtney J. Kihlberg, MD, MSPH[b],
Sarah E. Taylor, DO[a]

KEYWORDS

- Elderly • Geriatric • Prevention • Screening • Counseling
- USPSTF

The geriatric population in the United States, defined as individuals ≥65 years of age, is increasing in size. Between 1989 and 2010, it rose from 25 to 40 million. It is expected to grow to almost 90 million in 2050.[1] The leading causes of death among this population include cardiovascular disease, cancer, diabetes, vaccine-preventable diseases, and unintentional injury. Morbidity and mortality from these causes can be improved by primary, secondary, and tertiary prevention efforts. As such, this article presents an evidence-based review of prevention modalities for common diseases in the elderly.

HEALTHY BEHAVIOR
Tobacco Cessation

Despite decades of clinical and public health measures to encourage all Americans to avoid the use of tobacco, 9% (95% confidence interval [CI], 7.8%–10.2%) of those over the age of 65 currently smoke.[2] The prevalence of this unhealthy behavior in the elderly ranges from 4.2% in Utah to 18.0% Nevada.[2]

The Task Force on Community Preventive Services recommends evidence-based primary preventive strategies to reduce initiation of tobacco use among all age groups in the general population. This includes initiatives such as mass media campaigns that are combined with other interventions and increasing the price of tobacco products.[3] The Task Force on Community Preventive Services also recommends secondary prevention modalities such as health care provider reminder systems to encourage patients to undertake cessation efforts, decreasing out-of-pocket cost for cessation therapies, and multifaceted cessation programs that include telephone

---

The authors have nothing to disclose.

[a] Department of Family and Community Medicine, Meharry Medical College, 1005 Dr D.B. Todd, Jr, Boulevard, Old Hospital, 3rd Floor, Nashville, TN 37208, USA

[b] Department of Family and Community Medicine, Division of Preventive Medicine, Meharry Medical College, 1005 Dr D.B. Todd, Jr, Boulevard, Old Hospital, 2nd Floor, Nashville, TN 37208, USA

* Corresponding author.
E-mail address: rzoorob@mmc.edu

Clin Geriatr Med 27 (2011) 523–539
doi:10.1016/j.cger.2011.07.003
0749-0690/11/$ – see front matter © 2011 Elsevier Inc. All rights reserved.

geriatric.theclinics.com

support for those attempting to quit.[3,4] Furthermore, the United States Preventive Services Task Force (USPSTF) recommends that clinicians ask all adults about tobacco use and provide interventions for those who do use tobacco products.[5] Although primary and secondary preventive efforts exist that specifically target youth, racial/ethnic minorities, and women of reproductive age, far fewer resources have been developed with the goal of assisting elderly individuals in tobacco cessation efforts. In 2009, the US Centers for Disease Control and Prevention (CDC), American Association of Retired Persons, and American Medical Association issued a report entitled *Promoting Preventive Services in Adults Age 50–64*, which does include tobacco cessation as a priority. One of the 6 calls to action emphasized in the report is to "expand tobacco cessation programs and policies" by addressing the need for insurance plans to cover cessation counseling and medications and for public health and medical professionals to adhere to evidence-based strategies such as those outlined by The Task Force on Community Preventive Services and the USPSTF.[6]

Nutrition

Although the general population in the United States is experiencing an obesity epidemic that is taking a significant toll on American's quality of life,[7] it is critical to remember that among the geriatric population, both extremes of excess caloric intake and inadequate nutrition must be prevented and treated. The prevalence of obesity (body mass index ≥ 30 kg/m^2) among elderly Americans is 23% (95% CI, 21.1%–25.0%), with the extremes of this range noted outside the continental United States (14.8% in Hawaii to 33.4% in Alaska).[2] Adequate consumption of fruits and vegetables is important to avoid weight excess and to maintain proper nutrition. Only 28.1% (95% CI, 24.9%–31.2%; range of 19.2% in Mississippi to 37% in Hawaii) of Americans greater than 65 years old eat greater than or equal to 5 servings of fruits and vegetables on a daily basis.[2] Although screening all adults for obesity is recommended, the USPSTF found insufficient evidence to recommend that medical providers routinely counsel all patients on proper nutrition.[5] The USPSTF does encourage intensive behavioral counseling to promote a healthy diet and encourage weight loss among obese individuals.[5]

On the other end of the weight spectrum, maintenance of adequate muscle mass and micronutrients, especially vitamins B$_{12}$ and D, are essential in preventing dementia, falls, osteoporosis, and multiple other conditions discussed throughout this review.[8–12] The article, Diets for Successful Aging, discusses nutrition in more detail.

Physical Activity

The importance of regular physical activity cannot be overemphasized in health maintenance and disease prevention. As such, it was 1 of the 10 leading health indicators in *Healthy People 2010* that remains on the proposed list for *Healthy People 2020*.[13,14] Furthermore, it is 1 of the 6 calls to action in the CDC's *Promoting Preventive Services for Adults 50–64*.[6]

In 2007, however, the CDC found that among elderly Americans, 32.5% (95% CI, 29.8%–35.1%; range from 23.2% in Hawaii to 44.8% in Kentucky) had no leisure time physical activity in the month preceding their inquiry.[2] Others have found far higher rates of inactivity, reporting that 66% to 75% of individuals greater than 75 years of age participate in no regular physical activity.[15]

The USPSTF determined that there is insufficient evidence to recommend routine behavioral counseling in a primary care setting to promote physical activity.[5] However, multiple other organizations have issued and/or support evidence-based guidelines for specific durations and intensities of physical activity. *The 2008 Physical Activity Guidelines for Adults* issued by the US Department of Health and Human

Services recommends 150 minutes of moderate physical activity or 75 minutes of vigorous activity weekly in addition to muscle strengthening activities greater than or equal to 2 days per week. These US Department of Health and Human Services guidelines specifically state that adults over the age of 65 should follow these same recommendations, as able, but with a special emphasis on improving balance to minimize the risk of falls.[16] Recommendations in 2007 from the American Heart Association and the American College of Sports Medicine are similar to the US Department of Health and Human Services recommendations regarding total duration of physical activity per week, but are more specific regarding how frequently activity should be performed throughout the week. They state that adults between the ages of 18 and 65 should have 30 minutes of moderate aerobic activity 5 days per week or 20 minutes of vigorous activity 3 days per week. Unfortunately, these recommendations do not specifically include elderly adults over the age of 65.[17]

Sleep

Approximately one half of older adults have difficulties falling and/or staying asleep.[18] Poor quality sleep among older adults has been associated with a multitude of underlying medical conditions, including obstructive sleep apnea, restless leg syndrome, and depression.[19,20] Furthermore, healthy older adults without signs or symptoms of obstructive sleep apnea have been found to experience more respiratory disturbances than younger individuals.[21] Difficulty sleeping may also be the result of age-related changes in circadian rhythms. Many elderly individuals experience advanced sleep phase, in which they go to bed earlier and wake up earlier than they did in their younger years. Although not pathologic itself, extreme changes can dramatically reduce quality of life.[19] If any of these conditions are left untreated, a lack of sleep and poor sleep quality can contribute to cardiovascular and psychiatric morbidity and mortality, frailty, an increased risk of falls, and additional risk for polypharmacy when medicinal sleep aids are sought.[19,22–24]

The USPSTF has no guidelines regarding the appropriate length of time the general public should sleep. However, the rationale behind recommendations for obesity screening and counseling does include considerations for sleep apnea.[5] The American Academy of Sleep Medicine and others recommend that adults, including elderly adults, get between 7 and 9 hours of sleep every night.[19,25] Among the elderly, emphasis on proper sleep hygiene is especially important and consideration should be given to such issues as establishing a consistent bedtime, limiting naps to 1 hour, avoiding caffeine and alcohol, and exposure to light during the day and darkness at bedtime.[19]

METABOLIC DISORDERS
Diabetes Mellitus

Sixteen million people are diagnosed with diabetes mellitus in the United States, with 90% of cases classified as type 2.[26] Additionally an estimated 8 million people are currently diabetic but remain undiagnosed.[26] Because the prevalence of diabetes increases with age, its impact on the elderly population is significant. An estimated 18% to 20% of people over age 65 are affected.[26] Diabetes-related morbidity and mortality are especially high among the elderly, with up to 20% experiencing macrovascular complications (eg, myocardial infarction) and 9% microvascular complications (eg, retinopathy, nephropathy).[27] In fact, diabetes is the most frequent cause of blindness and end-stage renal disease in the United States, the rates of which increase with the duration of disease and with poor glycemic control.[27]

The USPSTF recommends screening for type 2 diabetes in asymptomatic adults with sustained hypertension (HTN; >135/80 mmHg), but found insufficient evidence for screening in normotensive, asymptomatic adults.[5] The American Diabetes Association (ADA) recommends screening asymptomatic individuals greater than or equal to 45 years of age for diabetes and repeating the screening every 3 years if results are normal. For overweight (body mass index ≥25) adults with greater than or equal to 1 risk factors, such as a personal history of gestational diabetes, family history of diabetes, HTN, hyperlipidemia, or for a member of a high-risk ethnic group, the ADA recommends screening at any age in adulthood, with a similar schedule of repeated screening every 3 years when normal.[28,29]

Among those diagnosed with diabetes, recommendations also exist regarding screening for diabetes-related complications. Data from the CDC indicated that in 2008, 28.5% of Americans over 40 years old had diabetic retinopathy. In over 4% of these cases, it was severe enough to lead to severe loss of vision.[30] Because diabetic retinopathy is the most common preventable causes of blindness in the United States, early detection and treatment are essential. The ADA recommends that all type 2 diabetics undergo a dilated eye examination by an ophthalmologist or optometrist at the time of diagnosis with repeat screens conducted annually, although less than 50% of the US diabetic population currently meets these guidelines.[30,31]

Although less prevalent than retinopathy at the time of diagnosis, diabetic nephropathy (prevalence of 7%) also represents a complication for which screening and treatment guidelines are available. The ADA recommends annual testing for urine albumin excretion and serum creatinine; and adequate blood pressure control using lifestyle modifications and a pharmacologic regimen including either angiotensin-converting enzyme inhibitors or angiotensin receptor blockers.[31]

To prevent complications of diabetic neuropathy, recommendations include annual screening for distal peripheral neuropathy using pinprick, 10-g monofilament pressure sensation, and/or vibration perception. Furthermore, all diabetics' feet should be examined for lesions and deformities, and footwear should be assessed at each visit.[31]

Of special note when treating elderly diabetics is the 2-fold risk of hypoglycemic episodes compared with younger patients. Whereas a hemoglobin A1c level of less than 7% is the recommended goal in all age groups, special care must be taken in the management of elderly individuals to avoid hypoglycemic episodes that could predispose them to falls and subsequent injury.[27]

Hyperlipidemia

Among American adults over the age of 20, the prevalence of high cholesterol (≥240 mg/dL) is approximately 18%. The prevalence is even higher among older adults aged 65 to 74 years, at 22% for men and 39% for women. Over the age of 75, the gender-specific prevalence rates are 14% for mean and 32% for women.[32] The connection between hyperlipidemia and cardiovascular disease is significant; however, the relative risk of high cholesterol to cardiovascular disease is not as daunting in the elderly as in the general population.[33]

The USPSTF recommends screening men age greater than or equal to 35 years and women age greater than or equal to 45 years for lipid disorders.[5] Among the elderly, 93.7% (95% CI, 92.3%–95.1%) have had their cholesterol checked within the preceding 5 years.[2]

Once diagnosed, additional considerations are used to guide treatment goals to prevent subsequent morbidity and mortality. Aggressive treatment for patients with known coronary heart disease (CHD) includes a low-density lipoprotein goal of less than or equal to 100 mg/dL.[34] For patients greater than 75 years old, more consideration to comorbidities, physiologic age, and health status must be considered.[33]

Hypothyroidism

The prevalence of hypothyroidism increases with age, but this condition is often overlooked in the elderly, in part because many individuals in this age group frequently report overlapping symptoms such as constipation and fatigue.[35] Women are affected more frequently than men. The most frequent underlying causes include autoimmune thyroiditis (57%) and postoperative complications (32%).[36] At this time, the USPSTF does not recommend routine screening with thyroid-stimulating hormone testing in asymptomatic individuals. In addition to typical hypothyroid symptoms such as weakness, fatigue, dry skin or hair, constipation, weight gain, cold intolerance, muscle cramps, edema of the face, hearing loss, and slow reflexes, it is important to have a high index of suspicion and initiate screening in the elderly with mental status changes, diastolic HTN, and/or bradycardia.[36]

Preventing treatment-related morbidity is also important because the prevalence of myxedema coma, and intraoperative and postoperative complications is higher among this age group. Because of the greater risk of cardiovascular intolerance to levothyroxine sodium, treatment should be initiated at lower doses in the elderly, with increases of 12.5 to 25 μg at 4- to 6-week intervals until optimal effect is achieved.[36]

CARDIOVASCULAR DISEASE
Coronary Heart and Cerebrovascular Disease

CHD is the overall leading cause of death in the United States, and is the leading cause of death among the elderly over the age of 65 years. Cerebrovascular accidents are the third leading cause of death overall, as well as the third leading cause among those over the age of 65.[37] The third report of the Expert Panel on Detection, Evaluation, and Treatment of High Blood Cholesterol in Adults includes on-line risk calculators that enable clinicians to easily determine a patient's 10-year risk for CHD.[34] Components included in the algorithm's calculation, including age, gender, smoking status, blood pressure, and total and high-density lipoprotein cholesterol levels, were derived from the Framingham Heart Study. Patients with a 10-year risk of less than 10% are considered low risk, and the USPSTF recommends against routine screening using modalities such as exercise stress tests, high sensitivity C Reactive Protein (hs-CRP) measurements, or computed tomography for coronary calcium in this group.[5,38] Furthermore, evidence is insufficient that these screening modalities are beneficial for asymptomatic patients at increased risk of CHD.[5,38]

Aspirin chemoprevention to prevent the development of CHD and cerebrovascular accidents, however, is strongly recommended by the USPSTF, as long as the potential benefits outweigh the risks, most notably of which is gastrointestinal bleeding. For men, low-dose aspirin is recommended from age 45 to 79 to reduce the risk of myocardial infarction, with studies documenting a 32% relative reduction in risk. For women, chemoprevention is recommended between the ages of 55 and 79 to reduce the risk of ischemic stroke, with a relative risk reduction of 17%.[5] Recent economic analyses also indicate that adherence to these guidelines could provide cost savings to both patients and the health care system through significant reductions in morbidity and mortality.[39] Studies have not shown a benefit of primary prevention for strokes in men or for CHD among women. Insufficient evidence currently exists to extend this recommendation beyond the age of 80 among either gender.[5]

HTN

HTN is a significant risk factor for morbidity and mortality from coronary artery disease, stroke, renal insufficiency, and dementia in the elderly.[40] Because individuals may remain asymptomatic, and the benefits of treatment often significantly outweigh any risks, the USPSTF strongly recommends that all adults over the age of 18 be screened.[5] The National Heart Lung and Blood Institute's Joint National Committee on Prevention, Detection, Evaluation, and Treatment of High Blood Pressure outlines considerations for treatment when HTN exists. Nonpharmacologic options both to prevent and limit HTN include smoking cessation, limiting alcohol consumption, maintenance of a healthy weight, active lifestyle, and balanced diet with adequate fruits, vegetables, and low-fat dairy products as well as limited fats and sodium.[5,40,41] Once present in the elderly, pharmacologic treatment is often necessary and frequently requires greater than or equal to 2 classes of medications.[40]

Abdominal Aortic Aneurysm

The greatest risk associated with abdominal aortic aneurysms (AAA) is acute rupture, which is fatal in 75% to 90% of occurrences.[5] The USPSTF currently recommends 1-time screening using ultrasonography in men 65 to 75 years old who have ever smoked. Although surgical repair of an AAA does present significant risk, among this population repair of aneurysms greater than 5.5 cm in diameter has been proven to decrease AAA-associated mortality. Although men greater than 75 years old are at greater risk for AAAs, the benefits of screening are limited because of their limited life expectancy and the prevalence of comorbidities that may limit successful outcomes from operative repair. The USPSTF recommends against screening in asymptomatic women of the same age, regardless of smoking history, largely because there is a substantially lower prevalence of large aneurysms among women.[5]

CANCERS
Colorectal Cancer

Colorectal cancer is third most common cancer in the United States and the third leading cause of cancer death.[42] Most colon cancer arises from adenomatous polyps, the incidence of which is known to increase with age.[43]

The evidence is conflicting regarding primary prevention of colon cancer. Studies of red meat consumption and cancer incidence are contradictory.[44] Although high fat intake does not increase the risk of colon cancer, there is an association with increasing adenomatous polyps.[44] Fiber intake and supplementation alone do not decrease the incidence of adenomatous polyps, although high-fiber foods such as fresh fruits and vegetables may be beneficial.[44-46] Results from a large cohort (452,755 patients) enrolled in the European Prospective Investigation into Cancer and Nutrition, who completed a dietary questionnaire between 1992 and 2000 and were followed for cancer until 2006, showed that high consumption of fruits and vegetables is associated with a decreased risk of colon cancer.[47]

The USPSTF recommends screening for colon cancer among average-risk individuals starting at age 50 and continuing until age 75. There is convincing evidence that screening this age group using fecal occult blood testing, sigmoidoscopy, or colonoscopy reduces mortality for colorectal cancer. Colonoscopy remains the gold standard for screening.[5] Despite these recommendations, only 67.6% of elderly Americans (95% CI, 65.1%–70.0%; range of 59.6% in Mississippi to 78.1% in the District of Columbia) undergo appropriate colon cancer screening.[2]

Use of both brochure reminders and telephone counseling has been shown to increase screening rates among minority populations.[48] The USPSTF also recommends against routine screening above age 75 because benefits of screening do not outweigh the harms.[5]

The American College of Gastroenterology also recommends that screening begin at age 50 for average-risk individuals. Since 2000, the American College of

Gastroenterology has clearly stated that colonoscopy every 10 years is the preferred screening method.[49]

Prostate Cancer

Prostate cancer accounts for approximately one third of new cancer cases in men, but only 10% of male cancer deaths.[50] Age is a significant risk factor for prostate cancer, with a lifetime prevalence of 30% among 50-year-old men and greater than 50% among 80-year-olds.[50] Although measurement of serum prostate-specific antigen has improved detection of prostate cancer, it is uncertain that this marker should be used for routine screening. Because the majority of men with prostate cancer do not die as a direct result of this malignancy, overdetection of benign and malignant disease followed by procedures in which the risk–benefit ratio is potentially unfavorable limits the utility of serum prostate-specific antigen screening.[50] As such, the USPTSF reports that there is insufficient evidence to recommend for or against prostate cancer screening in men less than 75 years of age. Furthermore, they recommend against screening in men greater than 75 years old.[5] As such, clinicians must weigh each individual patient's history, signs, and symptoms when considering screening for prostate cancer.

Cervical Cancer

Although the incidence and mortality from cervical cancer have been declining because of improvements in primary prevention, screening, and treatment, cervical cancer still accounts for nearly 10% of cancer cases among women each year.[51] Although common behavioral risk factors for the disease decrease with age, 10% of all cervical cancer cases occur in women greater than 75 years old and the incidence over age 65 is 1.2 times that for 45- to 64-year-olds.[52] Furthermore, advanced age at time of diagnosis is an independent risk factor of poor prognosis.[53] Nonetheless, in consideration of all risks and benefits associated with screening, the USPSTF currently recommends that women older than age 65 cease screening if recent Pap smears have been normal and the patient is not at high risk. Other organizations (eg, American Cancer Society/American Geriatrics Society/American College of Obstetricians and Gynecologists) recommend screening stop at age 70. Furthermore, women who have had a hysterectomy for benign disease do not benefit from routine Pap smears.[5]

Breast Cancer

According to the National Cancer Institute, 1 in 8 women develops breast cancer during her lifetime. The age-specific distribution of breast cancer is as follows: Women between the ages of 55 and 64 account for approximately 21% of cases, ages 65 to 74 for 20%, ages 75 to 84 for 21%, and greater than 85 years for 15.1%.[54] The USPSTF recently modified its recommendations to include screening mammography every 2 years for all women ages 50 to 74.[5] Although screening among asymptomatic women before the age of 50 is not routinely recommended, consideration on a case-by-case basis for women with increased risk should involves shared decision making based on the patient's personal history, family history, and values.[5] The USPSTF also concluded that there is insufficient evidence at this time for routine screening mammography over the age of 75.[5] Furthermore, they recommend against breast self-examination as a reliable screening modality and have found insufficient evidence that clinical breast examinations are beneficial in women over age 40.[5] Aspects of these recommendations conflict with those issued by the American

Cancer Society, which state that women over age 40 should have annual clinical breast examinations and screening mammography. The American Cancer Society also supports breast self-examinations as an option for women beginning in their 20s. The CDC found that, among elderly women, 79.0% (95% CI, 76.1%–81.8%; range of 68.1% in Mississippi to 86.1% in Massachusetts) had obtained a mammogram in the last 2 years.[2]

IMMUNIZATIONS
Herpes Zoster (Shingles)

Shingles can occur in any individual previously exposed to the varicella zoster virus (chickenpox). It is more common in individuals over the age of 50 or those with comprised immune systems. Owing in part to the high lifetime prevalence of this condition (estimated to be 1 in 3), the intensity and longevity of pain that occurs with postherpetic neuralgia, and the potential for ocular involvement and blindness, a vaccine for shingles was developed. The single-dose zoster vaccine, which contains the same but higher concentration of the live virus strain as the varicella vaccination, is recommended at the age of 60.[55] It reduced the risk of shingles by approximately 50% during clinical trials, and also helped to decrease the intensity of pain in those who were affected.[56] Currently, CDC recommendations state that it is unnecessary to confirm, either through history or serologic testing, that a patient has been exposed to chickenpox in the past before the administration of the zoster vaccine.[55] The CDC has compiled multiple tools to assist clinicians in improving adult vaccination rates. These are available online from www.cdc.gov/vaccines/recs/rate-strategies/adultstrat.htm.

Influenza

Beginning with the 2010/2011 season, the CDC now recommends annual influenza vaccinations for everyone greater than 6 months of age.[55] The live virus, nasal spray preparations are not licensed for use in adults greater than or equal to 50 years old, so all elderly individuals should receive the trivalent inactivated vaccination administered intramuscularly. In fact, a high-dose formulation containing 60 μg each of the 3 strains per 0.5-mL dose has been licensed for individuals greater than or equal to 65 years of age.[55] The Advisory Committee on Immunization Practices notes the availability of high-dose vaccine for the 2010/2011influenza season and that a study is under way to evaluate the relative effectiveness of high-dose vaccine compared with the standard dose.

Among the elderly, 72% (95% CI, 70.8%–73.3%; range from 60.2% in the District of Columbia to 80% in Rhode Island) had received a flu vaccine in the last year.[2] Although this statistic is admirable, adults over the age of 65 years have accounted for 70% to 90% of the mortality associated with this virus in the last 30 years.[57]

Pneumococcal

Streptococcus pneumoniae infection can cause pneumonia, meningitis, and bacteremia, and elderly individuals are at greater risk for morbidity and mortality than younger adults. Primary prevention includes 1 dose of pneumococcal polysaccharide vaccination (as opposed to the conjugate formulation given to young children) for all adults age greater than or equal to 65 years. This vaccination is also recommended for children and adults ages 2 to 64 years of age with certain chronic medical conditions or immune deficiencies. For elderly adults who did receive a dose before age 65, a second dose should be given after the 65th birthday and greater than or equal to 5 years after the first dose.[55] It is estimated that this vaccination has reduced the risk of pneumonia among elderly Americans by 44% to 61%.[58] The CDC found that among this population, 67.3% (95% CI, 64.4%–70.1%; range from 55.9% in the District of Columbia to 74.0% in Oregon) had ever received a pneumonia vaccine.[2]

Other Immunizations: Tdap, Meningococcal, and Hepatitis

All adults should have completed a primary series of tetanus and diphtheria (Td) vaccination. If incomplete, a 3-dose series spaced over a 7-month timeframe is advised (a 3-dose series is recommended only if no primary shots were given). After the primary series, booster doses should be administered every 10 years, even into the latest stage of life. To combat a rise in pertussis (whooping cough) cases, current Advisory Committee on Immunization Practices guidelines also recommend that greater than or equal to 1 dose in the primary adult series or among the booster doses include acellular pertussis (Tdap).[55] Tdap is not approved for those greater than 64 years of age.

Vaccination against *Neisseria meningitidis,* hepatitis A, and hepatitis B are also appropriate for certain populations of elderly individuals, including those with medical, occupational, and lifestyle risk factors.[55]

MENTAL HEALTH
Depression

Most large-scale studies estimate the prevalence of depression among community-dwelling adults greater than or equal to 65 years to be 1% to 5%.[59] Depression in older adults is usually undetected or diagnosed late, which is unfortunate; morbidity and mortality form late-life depression is higher than for younger adults owing to comorbid conditions and a higher incidence of suicide.[60,61]

Prevention efforts should be targeted at patients with increased risk with special emphasis on recognizing and treating older adults with subsyndromic symptoms to prevent major depressive episodes.[62] Other primary preventive strategies include early recognition and pharmacologic or counseling treatment of sleep disorders, bereavement, and comorbid medical conditions. Additionally, programs to educate older adults about symptoms of depression may be beneficial.[62]

The initial guidelines to screen for depression were produced by the Agency for Healthcare Research and Quality in 1993. Although they did not specifically target older adults, the guidelines are still pertinent. The USPSTF recommends screening adults for depression when staff-assisted depression care supports are in place to ensure accurate diagnosis, effective treatment, and follow-up. The USPTF recommends against routinely screening adults for depression when staff-assisted depression care supports are not in place.[5] There are many formal tools to screen for depression in older adults, although the most practical method uses the following 2 questions: (1) Over the past 2 weeks have you felt depressed, down, or hopeless? and (2) Over the past 2 weeks have you felt a decrease in pleasure or interest in doing things?[5]

The American Academy of Family Physicians recommends screening for depression in adults and follows the USPSTF recommendations.[63]

MUSCULOSKELETAL
Osteoporosis and Prevention of Falls

Osteoporosis affects 10 million people in the United States, with women over the age of 50 accounting for 1 to 4 million of those cases.[64] The prevalence among those over the age of 60 is estimated to be 30% to 40%. Furthermore, 14 million more people have low bone mass. As such, osteoporosis is a significant risk factor for potential morbidity and mortality, especially among elderly individuals who sustain a fall. An estimated 30% of adults over age 70 sustain greater than or equal to 1 fall. Approximately 3% to 4% of those who fall sustain a fracture and the relative risk of fracture increases with the number of risk factors for falling (eg, visual impairment, cognitive impairment, weakness, poor balance, chronic illness, polypharmacy).[65] The lifetime risk for osteoporotic fractures is currently estimated at 50% in women and 20% in men.[65] Hip fractures, the most serious type of all fall-related fractures, are a major contributor to death, disability, and diminished quality of life among older adults.[66] Rates of hospitalization for hip fractures for Americans over the age of 65 are 1026 per 100,000 women and 458 per 100,000 men.[2]

Screening and prevention can significantly reduce morbidity, mortality, and costs associated with osteoporosis and falls. Risk factors for osteoporosis are multifactorial and include female gender, Asian or white race, increased age, postmenopausal status, a history of certain medications (eg, steroids, antipsychotics), and family history. Lifestyle choices contribute significantly to risk as well, with smoking, alcohol use, poor nutrition, and a lack of weight-bearing exercise all increasing an individual's risk.[67] The Aerobics Center Longitudinal Study found an increase in walking-related falls among physically inactive elderly men among participants.[68]

The USPSTF currently recommends routine osteoporosis screening for women ≥65 and for those at increased risk beginning at age 60 using bone mineral density screening, typically conducted with dual energy x-ray absorptiometry scanning.[5] The American College of Preventive Medicine Prevention Practice Committee also advocates for screening in men over the age of 70 years and in younger men and women with risk factors, which can be assessed using existing osteoporosis risk assessment tools.[69] Determination of increased risk may be based on height loss, kyphosis, history of fractures, long-term steroid use, or prior abnormalities on bone mineral density testing.[65,67]

The cornerstones of prevention and early treatment of osteoporosis include weight-bearing exercise and adequate calcium and vitamin D intake, as discussed in the article, "Aging and the Effects of Vitamins and Supplements." Bisphosphonates are the now the favored pharmacologic tool; hormone replacement therapy has become less common. Addressing and modifying risk factors for falls can also greatly improve morbidity and mortality among the elderly, and should be considered first-line therapy.[8,65]

PROMOTING INDEPENDENCE
Hearing Loss

The 2003 and 2004 National Health and Nutrition Examination Survey found that 16.1% of the adult population (ages 20–69) had speech frequency hearing loss, with a prevalence of greater than 50% among individuals over age 75.[70] The National Health and Nutrition Examination Survey also showed that smoking, noise exposure, and cardiovascular risk factors result in hearing loss at an earlier age. Therefore, primary prevention of hearing loss should start well before the age of 65, and even as young as adolescence.[70]

Screening using a whispered voice test is both sensitive and specific; however, pure tone audiometry is the gold standard.[71] The USPSTF is currently updating its 1996 recommendations regarding screening in the elderly.[5] The American Geriatrics Society recommends annual evaluation of the elderly using the screening version of the Hearing Handicap Inventory for the Elderly, a 10-item questionnaire to evaluate for a functional decline in hearing or a hearing handicap, with or without handheld audiometry.[72]

Visual Acuity

Vision loss is also very common in older adults. In 2000, it was estimated that 1.8 million older adults had a vision impairment.[73] The USPSTF concludes that the current evidence is insufficient to assess the balance of benefits and harms of screening for visual acuity for the improvement of outcomes in older adults in the primary care setting.[5] Similarly, there is insufficient evidence for routinely screening adults for glaucoma, and studies have reported very low yield when such screening has been implemented.[5,74] The USPSTF did find, however, that early treatment of age-related macular degeneration, cataracts, and refractive errors improves the loss of visual acuity.[5]

Other societies have more specific recommendations, many of which are based solely on expert consensus or descriptive studies. The American Academy of Ophthalmology recommends that older adults receive a comprehensive eye examination every 1 to 2 years.[75] The Canadian Task Force on Periodic Health Examination states that visual acuity screening should be part of the physical examination for adults greater than 65 years of age.[76]

Driver Safety

The elderly are more prone to motor vehicle collisions, owing in part to visual, motor, and functional impairments.[77] To prevent accidents, many states have implemented stringent visual checks for elderly. In Florida, for example, stricter visual acuity screening for drivers greater than 80 years of age has resulted in a decrease in car accident death rates for that age group.[78] Some countries require a comprehensive assessment of individuals over age 75 by primary care physicians to improve driver safety.[79] Furthermore, cognitive problems can impair an elderly individual's ability to drive. A multidisciplinary, comprehensive assessment of older, cognitively impaired drivers seems to be the best way to enhance public and personal safety related to driving.[80] The American Academy of Neurology has issued guidelines for patients based on the level of dementia.[81] One specific component is to use simulators to actively train elderly drivers to negotiate intersections. Younger drivers tend to scan intersections more effectively while making a turn; active training of the elderly improves the ability to turn more effectively and safely.[82]

Incontinence

Urinary incontinence is defined as the involuntary leakage of urine. It is common in the geriatric population, affecting 1 out of 3 older women, and may significant reduce quality of life.[83] A longitudinal study in Australia that utilized multiple surveys from a large cohort of older women showed a strong association between incontinence and abnormal body mass index, dysuria, and constipation, thereby identifying multiple opportunities for prevention in elderly women.[84]

The American Geriatric Society recommends that clinicians document the presence or absence of incontinence in the initial evaluation of the vulnerable elderly. It also recommends to rescreen every 2 years, with special consideration for the impact incontinence may have on the patient's quality of life. Although there is no clear evidence that this practice improves treatment, many elderly individuals will not report incontinence unless specifically asked. Screening may thereby foster timely detection and treatment.[85]

Preventing Abuse and Neglect

Although the scope of this article does not allow adequate room for a complete discussion of this topic, it is critical to acknowledge the importance of preventing elder abuse and neglect. Clinicians should be aware that maltreatment of the elderly can occur through physical violence, neglect, emotional abuse, and financial exploitation. Assessing caregivers for burnout, discussing legal matters such as living wills and advanced directives, and obtaining social services for patients are all important measures in preventing elder abuse and neglect.

AVOIDING ADVERSE EFFECTS FROM POLYPHARMACY

According to the US Census Bureau, individuals greater than 65 years of age account for 12% of the population, but consume 32% of prescriptions. There are many definitions of polypharmacy, but most simply stated, it is the use of more medications than is clinically necessary. For every elderly patient, it is essential to answer the question, "Is every drug clinically indicated for this unique patient and prescribed at its lowest effective dose?" If the answer is no, polypharmacy exists. Polypharmacy leads to adverse drug events, decreased adherence to drug regimens, poor quality of life, and unnecessary drug expenses.[86] Furthermore, the use of greater than 6 drugs may be an independent predictor of increased mortality in the geriatric patient.[87]

Primary prevention should include screening all elderly patients for the number, type, and necessity of medications they are taking. At least yearly, and more often if indicated, conduct an "annual brown bag inspection" by asking patients to bring in all medications including prescription, over-the-counter, vitamin, and herbal preparations. Discuss all of the medications with the elderly patient and care provider and plan a drug reduction strategy.[88] This process involves the following 5 steps: Assessing the total number and type of medications, reviewing for possible interactions, minimizing nonessential medications, gradual optimization (ie, do not make all changes simultaneously), and reassessing at each subsequent visit.[88]

Special consideration should be given to medications that are typically inappropriate for use in the elderly population. These include, but are not limited to, propoxyphene, muscle relaxants, antispasmodics/anticholinergics, diphenhydramine, amitriptyline, amiodarone, long-acting benzodiazepines, and mepiridne.[89,90]

SUMMARY

The management of the medical, psychological, and social conditions affecting elderly individuals can be extremely complex owing to the high prevalence of multiple comorbidities. It is essential for clinicians and public health professionals to remember that preventive measures should remain a priority even as patients enter later stages of life. Primary prevention through such modalities as immunizations and counseling, secondary prevention via screening and early detection, and tertiary prevention of associated morbidity and mortality through proper disease management are critical to enable elderly patients to maintain the highest possible quality of life. Provision of these services should be a priority in both the one-on-one, clinic-based setting and through community-wide initiatives, 1 example of which is the Sickness Prevention Achieved through Regional Collaboration (SPARC) model.[91]

REFERENCES

1. National population projections. 2008. Available at: http://www.census.gov/population/www/projections/summarytables.html. Accessed October, 2010.

2. The state of aging and health in America report. 2007. Available at: http://apps. nccd.cdc.gov/SAHA/Default/IndicatorMenu.aspx.

3. The guide to community preventive services. 2010. Available at: http://www. thecommunityguide.org/index.html. Accessed September, 2010.

4. Ranney L, Melvin C, Lux L, et al. Tobacco use: prevention, cessation, and control. Evid Rep Technol Assess (Full Rep) 2006;140:1–120.

5. USPSTF Recommendations. Available at: http://www.uspreventiveservicestaskforce. org/uspstopics.htm#AZ. Accessed September, 2010.

6. Promoting preventive services for adults 50–64. Available at: http://apps.nccd. cdc.gov/DACH_PPS/Static/CallToAction.aspx. Accessed July 14, 2011.

7. Jia H, Lubetkin El. Obesity-related quality-adjusted life years lost in the U.S. from 1993 to 2008. Am J Prev Med 2010;39:220–7.

8. Kalyani RR, Stein B, Valiyil R, et al. Vitamin D treatment for the prevention of falls in older adults: systematic review and meta-analysis. J Am Geriatr Soc 2010;58:1299–310.

9. Ciaschini PM, Straus SE, Dolovich LR, et al. Community based intervention to optimize osteoporosis management: randomized controlled trial. BMC Geriatr 2010; 10:60.

10. Rao SS, Budhwar N, Ashfaque A. Osteoporosis in men. Am Fam Physician 2010;82: 503–8.

11. Buell JS, Dawson-Hughes B, Scott TM, et al. 25-Hydroxyvitamin D, dementia, and cerebrovascular pathology in elders receiving home services. Neurology 2010;74: 18–26.

12. Agriculture USDoHaHSaUSDo. Executive summary: dietary guidelines for Americans, 2005. Available at: http://www.health.gov/dietaryguidelines/dga2005/document/ html/executivesummary.htm. Accessed November, 2010.

13. Healthy people 2010. Available at: http://www.healthypeople.gov/2010. Accessed September, 2010.

14. Health indicators healthy people 2020. Available at: http://www.nevadapublic healthfoundation.org/health-indicators-healthy-people-2020.asp. Accessed September, 2010.

15. deJong AA, Franklin BA. Prescribing exercise for the elderly: current research and recommendations. Curr Sports Med Rep 2004;3:337–43.

16. 2008 physical activity guidelines for Americans. Available at: http://www.health.gov/ paguidelines/guidelines/default.aspx. Accessed September, 2010.

17. Haskell WL, Lee IM, Pate RR, et al. Physical activity and public health: updated recommendation for adults from the American College of Sports Medicine and the American Heart Association. Circulation 2007;116:1081–93.

18. Roepke SK, Ancoli-Israel S. Sleep disorders in the elderly. Indian J Med Res 2010; 131:302–10.

19. Sleep and growing older. Available at: http://www.sleepeducation.com/Topic.aspx? id=30. Accessed July 14, 2011.

20. Avidan AY. Sleep in the geriatric patient population. Semin Neurol 2005;25:52–63.

21. Pavlova MK, Duffy JF, Shea SA. Polysomnographic respiratory abnormalities in asymptomatic individuals. Sleep 2008;31:241–8.

22. Cherniack EP, Cherniack NS. Obstructive sleep apnea, metabolic syndrome, and age: will geriatricians be caught asleep on the job? Aging Clin Exp Res 2010;22:1–7.

23. Ensrud KE, Blackwell TL, Redline S, et al. Sleep disturbances and frailty status in older community-dwelling men. J Am Geriatr Soc 2009;57:2085–93.

24. Kuo HK, Yang CC, Yu YH, et al. Gender-specific association between self-reported sleep duration and falls in high-functioning older adults. J Gerontol A Biol Sci Med Sci 2010;65:190–6.

25. Reynolds CF 3rd, Serody L, Okun ML, et al. Protecting sleep, promoting health in later life: a randomized clinical trial. Psychosom Med 2010;72:178–86.

26. Florence JA, Yeager BF. Treatment of type 2 diabetes mellitus. Am Fam Physician 1999;59:2835–44.

27. Wallace JI. Management of diabetes in the elderly. Clinical Diabetes 1999;17.

28. Clinical practice recommendations 2005. Diabetes Care 2005;28(Suppl 1):S1–79.

29. Summary of revisions for the 2010 clinical practice recommendations. Diabetes Care 2010;33(Suppl 1):S3.

30. National Diabetes Fact Sheet, 2011. Available at: http://www.cdc.gov/diabetes/pubs/pdf/ndfs_2011.pdf. Accessed August, 2011.

31. Standards of medical care in diabetes—2010. Diabetes Care 2010;33(Suppl 1):S11–61.

32. Tanner M, Link N. Hyperlipidemia: part 1. Evaluation and dietary management. West J Med 2001;175:246–50.

33. Dalal D, Robbins JA. Management of hyperlipidemia in the elderly population: an evidence-based approach. South Med J 2002;95:1255–61.

34. Expert Panel on Detection, Evaluation, and Treatment of High Blood Cholesterol in Adults. ATP 3 guidelines 2001, reprinted 2010; NIH Publication number 02-3305. Available at: http://www.nhlbi.nih.gov/guidelines/cholesterol/index.htm links. Accessed October, 2010.

35. Adlin V. Subclinical hypothyroidism: deciding when to treat. Am Fam Physician 1998;57:776–80.

36. Jameson JL, Weetman AP. Disorders of the thyroid gland. In: Kasper DL, Fauci AS, Longo DL, et al, editors. Harrison's principles of internal medicine. 16th edition. New York: McGraw Hill; 2005. p. 2109–12.

37. Xu J, Kochanek KD, Murphy SL, et al. Deaths: final data for 2007. National Vital Statistics Reports 2010. Available at: http://www.cdc.gov/NCHS/data/nvsr/nvsr58/nvsr58_19.pdf. Accessed October, 2010.

38. Lim LS, Haq N, Mahmood S, et al. Atherosclerotic cardiovascular disease screening in adults: American College of Preventive Medicine position statement on preventive practice. Am J Prev Med 2011;40:381 e1–10.

39. Manson SC, Benedict A, Pan F, et al. Potential economic impact of increasing low dose aspirin usage on CVD in the US. Curr Med Res Opin 2010;26:2365–73.

40. Joint National Committee on Prevention, Detection, Evaluation, and Treatment of High Blood Pressure. Available at: www.nhlbi.nih.gov/guidelines/hypertension/jncintro.htm. Accessed October, 2010.

41. Kolasa KM. Dietary Approaches to Stop Hypertension (DASH) in clinical practice: a primary care experience. Clin Cardiol 1999;22(7 Suppl):III16–22.

42. Jemal A, Siegel R, Xu J, et al. Cancer statistics, 2010. CA Cancer J Clin 2010;60:277–300.

43. Patel BB, Yu Y, Du J, et al. Age-related increase in colorectal cancer stem cells in macroscopically normal mucosa of patients with adenomas: a risk factor for colon cancer. Biochem Biophys Res Commun 2009;378:344–7.

44. Wilkins T, Reynolds PL. Colorectal cancer: a summary of the evidence for screening and prevention. Am Fam Physician 2008;78:1385–92.

45. Food, nutrition, physical activity, and the prevention of cancer: a global perspective. 2007. Available at: http://www.wcrf.org/research/expert_report/recommendations.php. Accessed July 14, 2011.

46. Mason JB. Nutritional chemoprevention of colon cancer. Semin Gastrointest Dis 2002;13:143–53.
47. van Duijnhoven FJ, Bueno-De-Mesquita HB, Ferrari P, et al. Fruit, vegetables, and colorectal cancer risk: the European Prospective Investigation into Cancer and Nutrition. Am J Clin Nutr 2009;89:1441–52.
48. Walsh JM, Salazar R, Nguyen TT, et al. Healthy colon, healthy life: a novel colorectal cancer screening intervention. Am J Prev Med 2010;39:1–14.
49. Rex DK, Johnson DA, Anderson JC, et al. American College of Gastroenterology guidelines for colorectal cancer screening 2009 [corrected]. Am J Gastroenterol 2009;104:739–50.
50. Chodak G. Prostate cancer: epidemiology, screening, and biomarkers. Rev Urol 2006;8(Suppl 2):S3–8.
51. Franco EL, Duarte-Franco E, Ferenczy A. Cervical cancer: epidemiology, prevention and the role of human papillomavirus infection. CMAJ 2001;164:1017–25.
52. National Cancer Institute. SEER cancer statistics review. Available at: http://seer.cancer.gov/statfacts/html/cervix.html#incidence-mortality. Accessed August 6, 2011.
53. Foxx-Orenstein A. IBS—review and what's new. MedGenMed 2006;8:20.
54. National Cancer Institute. Breast cancer. 2010. Available at: http://www.cancer.gov/cancertopics/types/breast. Accessed July 14, 2011.
55. US Centers for Disease Control and Prevention. Advisory committee on immunization practices recommendations. Vaccines and preventable diseases. Available at: http://www.cdc.gov/vaccines/vpd-vac/default.htm. Accessed September 2010.
56. US Centers for Disease Control and Prevention. Shingles vaccine information sheet. http://www.cdc.gov/vaccines/pubs/vis/downloads/vis-shingles.pdf. Accessed January 2011.
57. Estimates of deaths associated with seasonal influenza—United States, 1976–2007. MMWR Morb Mortal Wkly Rep 2010;59:1057–62.
58. Fingar AR, Francis BJ. American College of Preventive Medicine practice policy statement: adult immunizations. Am J Prev Med 199814:156–8.
59. Hasin DS, Goodwin RD, Stinson FS, et al. Epidemiology of major depressive disorder: results from the National Epidemiologic Survey on Alcoholism and Related Conditions. Arch Gen Psychiatry 2005;62:1097–106.
60. Blazer DG. Depression in late life: review and commentary. J Gerontol A Biol Sci Med Sci 2003;58:249–65.
61. Klap R, Unroe KT, Unutzer J. Caring for mental illness in the United States: a focus on older adults. Am J Geriatr Psychiatry 2003;11:517–24.
62. Fiske A, Wetherell JL, Gatz M. Depression in older adults. Annu Rev Clin Psychol 2009;5:363–89.
63. American Academy of Family Physicians. AAFP clinical recommendations. Available at: http://www.aafp.org/online/en/home/clinical/clinicalrecs.html. Accessed October, 2010.
64. Iqbal MM. Osteoporosis: epidemiology, diagnosis, and treatment. South Med J 2000; 93:2–18.
65. Ullom-Minnich P. Prevention of osteoporosis and fractures. Am Fam Physician 1999;60:194–202.
66. Wolinsky FD, Fitzgerald JF, Stump TE. The effect of hip fracture on mortality, hospitalization, and functional status: a prospective study. Am J Public Health 1997;87:398–403.
67. National Osteoporosis Foundation. 2011. Available at: http://www.nof.org/. Accessed January, 2011.
68. Mertz KJ, Lee DC, Sui X, et al. Falls among adults: the association of cardiorespiratory fitness and physical activity with walking-related falls. Am J Prev Med 2010;39:15–24.

69. Lim LS, Hoeksema LJ, Sherin K. Screening for osteoporosis in the adult U.S. population: ACPM position statement on preventive practice. Am J Prev Med 2009;36:366–75.

70. Agrawal Y, Platz EA, Niparko JK. Prevalence of hearing loss and differences by demographic characteristics among US adults: data from the National Health and Nutrition Examination Survey, 1999-2004. Arch Intern Med 2008;168:1522–30.

71. Pirozzo S, Papinczak T, Glasziou P. Whispered voice test for screening for hearing impairment in adults and children: systematic review. BMJ 2003;327:967.

72. Yueh B, Shekelle P. Quality indicators for the care of hearing loss in vulnerable elders. J Am Geriatr Soc 2007;55(Suppl 2):S335–9.

73. Chou R, Dana T, Bougatsos C. Screening older adults for impaired visual acuity: a review of the evidence for the U.S. Preventive Services Task Force. Ann Intern Med 2009;151:44–58.

74. Stoutenbeek R, de Voogd S, Wolfs RC, et al. The additional yield of a periodic screening programme for open-angle glaucoma: a population-based comparison of incident glaucoma cases detected in regular ophthalmic care with cases detected during screening. Br J Ophthalmol 2008;92:1222–6.

75. American Academy of Ophthalmology. Preferred practice patterns. Available at: http://one.aao.org/ce/practiceguidelines/ppp_content.aspx?cid=64e9df91-dd10-4317-8142-6a87eee7f517. Accessed October, 2010.

76. Periodic health examination, 1995 update: 3. Screening for visual problems among elderly patients. Canadian Task Force on the Periodic Health Examination. CMAJ 1995;152:1211–22.

77. McGwin G Jr, Sims RV, Pulley L, et al. Relations among chronic medical conditions, medications, and automobile crashes in the elderly: a population-based case-control study. Am J Epidemiol 2000;152:424–31.

78. McGwin G Jr, Sarrels SA, Griffin R, et al. The impact of a vision screening law on older driver fatality rates. Arch Ophthalmol 2008;126:1544–7.

79. Kamenoff I. Assessing elderly people to drive—practical considerations. Aust Fam Physician 2008;37:727–32.

80. Carr DB, Ott BR. The older adult driver with cognitive impairment: "it's a very frustrating life." JAMA 2010;303:1632–41.

81. Dubinsky RM, Stein AC, Lyons K. Practice parameter: risk of driving and Alzheimer's disease (an evidence-based review): report of the quality standards subcommittee of the American Academy of Neurology. Neurology 2000;54:2205–211.

82. Romoser MR, Fisher DL. The effect of active versus passive training strategies on improving older drivers' scanning in intersections. Hum Factors 2009;51:652–68.

83. Goode PS, Burgio KL, Richter HE, et al. Incontinence in older women. JAMA 2010;303:2172–81.

84. Byles J, Millar CJ, Sibbritt DW, et al. Living with urinary incontinence: a longitudinal study of older women. Age Ageing 2009;38:333–8.

85. Fung CH, Spencer B, Eslami M, et al. Quality indicators for the screening and care of urinary incontinence in vulnerable elders. J Am Geriatr Soc 2007;55(Suppl 2):S443–9.

86. Cooper JW. Probable adverse drug reactions in a rural geriatric nursing home population: a four-year study. J Am Geriatr Soc 1996;44:194–7.

87. Incalzi RA, Gemma A, Capparella O, et al. Predicting mortality and length of stay of geriatric patients in an acute care general hospital. J Gerontol 1992;47:M35–9.

88. Cefalu C. Knowledge and participation in the care planning process by physicians in the nursing home setting: the case of falls. Annals Long-Term Care 2009;17:25–7.

89. Beers MH, Ouslander JG, Rollingher I, et al. Explicit criteria for determining inappropriate medication use in nursing home residents. UCLA Division of Geriatric Medicine. Arch Intern Med 1991;151:1825–32.

90. Fick DM, Cooper JW, Wade WE, et al. Updating the Beers criteria for potentially inappropriate medication use in older adults: results of a US consensus panel of experts. Arch Intern Med 2003;163:2716–24.

91. Shenson D, Benson W, Harris AC. Expanding the delivery of clinical preventive services through community collaboration: the SPARC model. Prev Chronic Dis 2008;5:A20.

Hormone Replacement Therapy in the Geriatric Patient: Current State of the Evidence and Questions for the Future. Estrogen, Progesterone, Testosterone, and Thyroid Hormone Augmentation in Geriatric Clinical Practice: Part 1

Erika Schwartz, MD[a],*, Kent Holtorf, MD[b]

KEYWORDS

- Hormone replacement • Estrogen • Progesterone
- Testosterone • Thyroid hormone • Bioidentical hormones

Geriatric medicine historically has been the domain of sick, frail, old, and aging populations of patients. Therapies for aging patients focus primarily on prolonging life, often at very high emotional and financial cost with little focus on the quality of life the patient experiences. As the proportion of aging people continues to rise, reducing the burden of age-related conditions becomes increasingly important in geriatric care. In addition, as the life expectancy of the population increases, years of disability follow unless comprehensive prevention and treatment of age-related diseases and frailty are addressed.

With the transition of the baby boomers into the geriatric population, a significant movement away from the disease-centric model and toward prevention and wellness maintenance and enhancement is taking place. The goal of this article is to present an up-to-date review of the literature on hormone augmentation in the elderly to help primary care physicians better evaluate and utilize hormone replacement and optimization strategies to benefit their patients. The scientific literature suggests that hormone supplementation with estrogen, progesterone, testosterone, growth hormone, and

[a] Age Management Institute, 200 West 57 Street, Suite 502, New York, NY 10019, USA
[b] Holtorf Medical Group, 23456 Hawthorne Boulevard, Suite 160, Torrance, CA 90505, USA
* Corresponding author.
E-mail address: Eschwartz@agemd.org

Clin Geriatr Med 27 (2011) 541–559
doi:10.1016/j.cger.2011.07.013
0749-0690/11/$ – see front matter © 2011 Elsevier Inc. All rights reserved.

geriatric.theclinics.com

support for menopausal and postmenopausal patients. As physicians become better informed about the available options of hormone therapies, the choices patients make will become truly informed and ultimately tailored to their individual needs.

If patients choose HRT, the US Preventive Services Task Force recommends that they use the smallest effective dose for the shortest possible time and that the patient see her doctor at least once a year to discuss whether she should stop and what new information may be available that might influence the patient's decision to stop or continue using hormones.[9] (An important note: As research continues, recommendations may change.) Of course, the patient may wish to continue regular breast cancer screenings, including annual physician breast exams and periodic mammograms. (ACOG recommends mammograms every 1–2 years during the 40s, and annually thereafter while the US Preventative Services Task Force recommends testing every 2 years starting only at the age of 50.)

As with most issues concerning health, the decision to use hormones is a personal one that ultimately must be made by the patient. It is the physician's role to help the patient make sure the decision is a well informed one with which the patient feels comfortable. The more knowledgeable and informed the physician is regarding the different types of hormone therapies available and the evidence supporting them, the more information he or she can provide for the patient. Before making a decision about HRT, women should consult with their physicians for individualized advice that takes into account types of hormone therapies available, recommendations of medical societies and governmental agencies, personal needs, and medical and family history.[2,10,11]

To help physicians better understand the state of the information as it relates to WHI and the conjugated equine estrogens and MPA, the findings of the WHI are recapped here. The results of the WHI indicated that if 10,000 women were given 0.625 mg of conjugated estrogen and 2.5 mg of medroxyprogesterone and followed for 5 years, there would be eight additional cases of breast cancer, seven additional coronary events, eight additional strokes, and eight additional cases of pulmonary embolism than in those women not receiving HRT. The major question, however, is: Would the results be different if different forms (synthetic vs. bioidentical) of HRT were used?

BIOIDENTICAL HORMONES

The WHI study did not evaluate other types of HRT; specifically, bioidentical or natural hormones. These are a class of hormones including estradiol, progesterone, and testosterone that are pharmaceutically indistinguishable from the same hormones naturally produced by the human body (as opposed to equine estrogens, which are the source of conjugated estrogens and are not a natural hormone combination for humans). Bioidentical or natural hormones have been used for decades in Europe and since the 1990s in the United States.[12–30]

Bioidentical Versus Synthetic

The molecular differences between bioidentical and nonhuman identical hormone preparations[31] are illustrated in **Fig. 1**.

State of the Evidence of Various Hormone Preparations in Women

The differences in action between conjugated equine estrogens, synthetic progestins, and bioidentical hormones have been described and studied extensively in the scientific literature over a period of 40 years.[32–35] Early small studies in the 1970s and

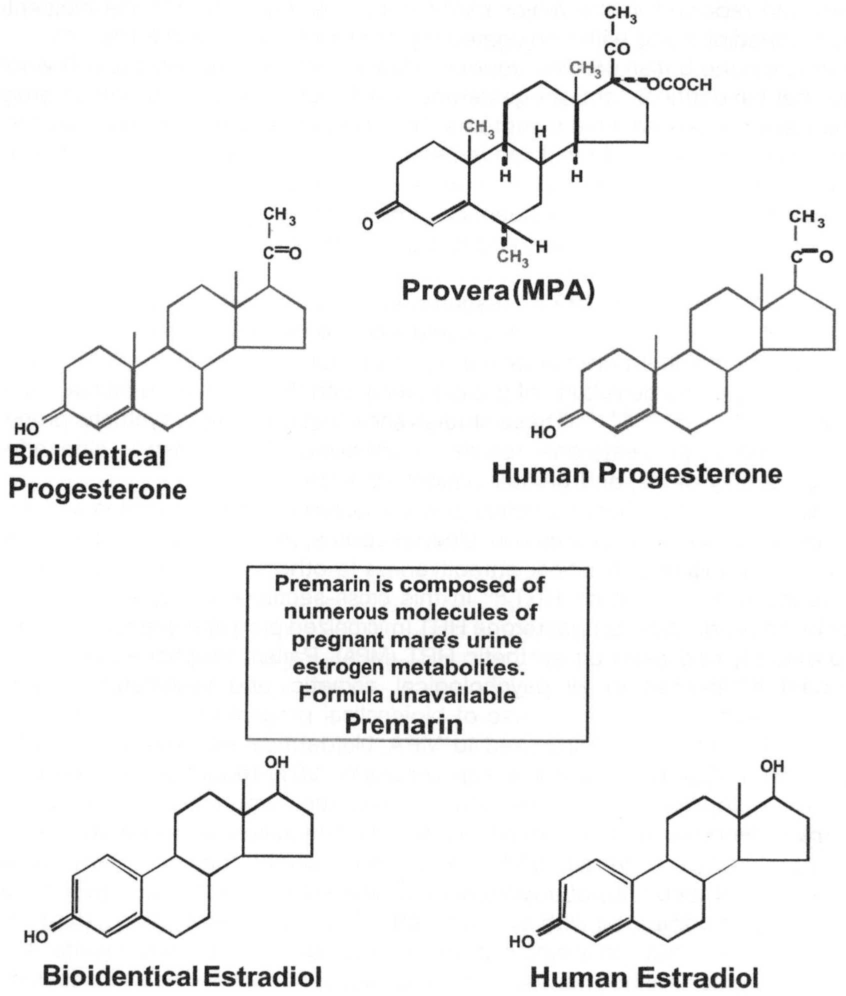

Fig. 1. The molecular formulas of various types of progestagens and estrogens. (*Adapted from* Schwartz E, Holtorf K. Prim Care Clin Office Pract 2008;35:669–705; with permission.)

1980s suggested the safety of bioidentical hormones, although the studies were too small to reach statistical significance.

As early as 1975, the safety of bioidentical estradiol appeared in the conventional medical literature.[20] Studies and reports of increased risk of endometrial and breast carcinoma among users of synthetic conjugated estrogens (the type of hormone preparations studied by the WHI) also appeared in the scientific literature in the 1970s.[19,36–38] By January 1978, the *Journal of the American Geriatrics Society* addressed the growing concern that treatment with exogenous synthetic estrogen could cause cancer and recommended the addition of a synthetically manufactured progestogen as a working solution.[39] Adding small doses of a progestogen (MPA) to either estradiol or conjugated estrogen (CEE) in a cycled manner was determined to be a safe solution to the carcinogenicity concern associated with the use of conjugated estrogens.[40]. It is noteworthy that in 1983, the options for treatment

Because the risks of synthetic progestins are now well established, further comparison studies between synthetic and bioidenticals would be unethical. Future research should be focused on bioidentical hormones versus placebo.

Cardiovascular: Bioidentical Progesterone Versus Synthetic Progestins

The only long-term study on myocardial infarction (MI) and stroke to date is the WHI, which did not address the effects of bioidentical hormones on cardiovascular events. In contrast, numerous studies including the WHI have found the use of a synthetic progestin will result in an increase in cardiovascular risk factors, including worsening of lipid profiles,[124-139] prevention of normal vasodilation and promotion of coronary artery vasospasm,[126,127,130,134,139] increasing hypercoagulability,[13,140,141] worsening insulin resistance,[132,142-144] and promotion of cardiovascular plaque formation.[131,135,137,138,145-147]

In addition, synthetic progestin is proven to increase the actual incidence of myocardial infarction and stroke.[2,139] Conversely, bioidentical progesterone has been shown *not* to have negative effects on the aforementioned cardiac risk factors in the short term in small studies. Unfortunately, these studies cannot be compared in scope and duration to the WHI study, leaving the question of whether bioidentical progesterone can actually protect from myocardial infarction or stroke in need of a more definitive answer.[23,124,129,133,136,148]

Cardiovascular Risk and Estrogen

The WHI Estrogen Alone trial differed from the better known WHI trial of estrogen plus progestin in that it enrolled women who did not have a uterus and did not need the progestin hormone supplementation to protect their endometrium from the well documented negative effects of conjugated equine estrogens. In the Estrogen Alone trial, 10,739 women with prior hysterectomy, aged 50 to 79 years, were assigned to take conjugated estrogens (Premarin) 0.625 mg daily or to placebo. The study was stopped ahead of schedule in February 2004 by the National Institutes of Health (NIH) because of increased stroke risk and a possible but not categorical increase incidence of myocardial infarction during the 7 years of follow-up. In addition, the conjugated estrogen studied in this arm of the WHI study did not prove to offer *any* overall protection against heart attack or coronary death in the hormone therapies studied.[149]

In conclusion, our extensive review of the literature finds that all hormones are not equal. Bioidentical and synthetic hormones have differing and often opposite effects. This is important because physicians are often exposed to confusing information about hormone replacement in general and have to help patients make safe and intelligent individual decisions.

Bioidentical hormones have been associated with patient satisfaction, symptom relief, improved cardiovascular risk factors, and reduced risk of breast cancer compared to their synthetic counterparts. Although more randomized control trials are needed to cement and clarify further the extent of the differences between bioidentical and synthetic hormones, the present authors believe that the current state of the evidence demonstrates that bioidentical hormones should be the preferred method of therapy when HRT is chosen. Further, physicians must become familiar and comfortable with the differences in the preparations of hormones available and adapt their prescribing practices accordingly.

TESTOSTERONE FOR WOMEN

Testosterone production in women derives from three sources: the ovaries, the adrenal glands, and from peripheral conversion from other circulating androgens.

Testosterone levels decrease with age, with levels in the fifth decade averaging about half of the level seen in women in their third decade.[150] This decline is due to a combination of factors: androgen production from the adrenal glands progressively declines with age and, although testosterone production from the ovaries remains relatively intact after menopause, the adrenal secretion of androstenedione declines by 50%.[150] The lower androstenedione levels result in a significant reduction in the peripheral conversion to testosterone at menopause. In addition, women who have undergone bilateral oophorectomy experience a 50% further reduction in testosterone levels.

Signs and symptoms of androgen insufficiency include loss of libido, fatigue, reduced sense of well-being, decreased lean body mass, and reduced bone density.[151]

Most commercial assays for the measurement of free and total testosterone levels were developed to measure the much higher levels in men. Consequently, assays in general lack the sensitivity and precision required to measure the normal low levels seen in women. Thus there is no real basis for most of the reference ranges used for testosterone measurements in women.[152,153] Also, serum levels have not been found to correlate with the presence or absence of symptoms (normal levels do not mean testosterone replacement will not be effective). Thus, if a normal testosterone level is found, it should not be used to rule out a deficiency in women or become the sole determinant when making the decision to treat or trying to make the connection between testosterone levels and symptomatology.

Although there is currently no FDA-approved testosterone preparation for the treatment of "testosterone insufficiency" in women, androgen replacement has been used off-label for more than 70 years.[154] Testosterone therapy in postmenopausal women has been shown to improve sexual desire and responsiveness,[155–158] sense of well-being,[159–162] and body composition[163,164] and to increase bone density.[157,165,166] All the studies reviewed in the preceding text are small with statistically significant results. However, more randomized control trials need to be performed to determine efficacy, optimal dosing, and risks.

Risks of Testosterone Treatment in Women

Several side effects are potentially associated with testosterone therapy in women, including potential adverse effects on the cardiovascular system, hirsutism, acne, and breast cancer.[167] The main concern with testosterone replacement in women is its potential negative effect on lipids. The use of testosterone has been shown in some studies to have significant adverse effect on lipid levels.[167,168] The findings include slight lowering of high-density lipoprotein but no appreciable effect on low-density lipoprotein.[168–170]

No randomized trials of sufficient size or duration have been reported to assess the breast cancer risk with testosterone replacement. Although no study reports significant increase in risk, we found two studies that in fact provide support for its use. A retrospective study by Dimitrakakis and colleagues in *Menopause* in 2004 found no increase in risk of breast cancer when adding testosterone to 508 women receiving conventional HRT, conventional synthetic HRT that were followed for an average of 5.8 years.[171] and the study by Hubayter and colleagues in *Climacteric* in 2008 showing positive results with testosterone usage for improvement of sexual dysfunction in postmenopausal women.[172]

Unwanted cosmetic effects, such as acne and hirsutism, are possible side effects associated with large doses of testosterone supplementation, especially in women with a history of such problems. If testosterone is given at an appropriate dose and closely monitored, these side effects tend to be minimal and resolve with a reduction in dose or discontinuation of therapy.[172]

25. Stahlberg C, Pedersen AT, Lynge E, et al. Increased risk of breast cancer following different regimens of hormone replacement therapy frequently used in Europe. Int J Cancer 2004;109:721–7.
26. Fournier A, Berrino F, Clavel-Chapelon F. Unequal risks for breast cancer associated with different hormone replacement therapies: results from the E3N cohort study. Breast Cancer Res Treat 2008;107:103–11.
27. Li CI, Malone KE, Porter PL, et al. Relationship between long durations and different regimens of hormone therapy and risk of breast cancer. JAMA 2003;289:3254–63.
28. Schindler AE. Differential effects of progestins. European Progestin Club. Maturitas 2003;46(Suppl 1):S3–5.
29. Montplaisir J, Lorrain J, Denesle R, et al. Sleep and menopause: differential effects of two forms of hormone replacement therapy. Menopause 2001;8:10–6.
30. Zegura B, Guzic-Salobir B, Sebestjen M, et al. The effects of various menopausal hormone therapies on markers of inflammation, coagulation, fibrinolysis, lipids and lipoproteins in healthy postmenopausal women. Menopause 2006;13:643–50.
31. Schwartz, E, Holtorf, K. Hormones in wellness and disease prevention: common practices, current state of the evidence, and questions for the future. Prim Care 2008;35:669–705.
32. Boothby LA, Doering PL, Kipersztok S. Bioidentical hormone therapy: a review. Menopause 2004;11:356–67.
33. Franke HR, Vermes I. Differential effects of progestogens on breast cancer cell lines. Maturitas 2003;46(Suppl 1):S55–8.
34. Druckmann R. Progestins and their effects on the breast. Maturitas 2003; 46(Suppl 1):S59–69.
35. Colditz G. Estrogen, estrogen plus progestin therapy and risk of breast cancer. Clin Cancer Res 2005;11(2 Pt 2):909s–17s.
36. Tourgeman DE, Gentzchein E, Stanczyk F, et al. Serum and tissue hormone levels of vaginally and orally administered estradiol. Am J Obtstet Gynecol 1999;180(6 Pt 1):1480–3.
37. Smith DC, Prentice R, Thompson DJ, et al. Association of exogenous estrogen and endometrial carcinoma. N Engl J Med 1975;293:1164–7.
38. Ziel HK, Finkle WD. Increased risk of endometrial carcinoma among users of conjugated estrogens. N Engl J Med 1975;293:1167–70.
39. Greenblatt RB, Stoddard LD. The estrogen-cancer controversy. J Am Geriatr Soc 1978;26:1–8.
40. Weiss N, Szekely D, Austin D. Increasing incidence of endometrial cancer in the United States. N Engl J Med 1976;294:1259–62.
41. Whitehead MI, Townsend PT, Gill DK, et al. Absorption and metabolism of oral progesterone. Br Med J 1980;280(6217):825–7.
42. Bergkvist L, Adami H, Persson I, et al. The risk of breast cancer after estrogen and estrogen-progestin replacement. N Engl J Med 1989;32:293–7.
43. Glass AG, Hoover RN. Rising incidence of breast cancer: relationship to stage and receptor status. J Natl Cancer Inst 1990;82:693–6.
44. Mack TM, Pike MC, Henderson BE, et al. Estrogens and endometrial cancer in a retirement community. N Engl J Med 1976;294:1262–7.
45. Foidart J, Colin C, Denoo X, et al. Estradiol and progesterone regulate the prolifer-ation of human breast epithelial cells. Fertil Steril 1998;69:963–9.
46. Maxson WS, Hargrove JT. Bioavailability of oral micronized progesterone. Fertil Steril 1985;44:622–6.
47. Whitehead MI, Fraser D, Schenkel L, et al. Transdermal administration of oestrogen/progesterone hormone replacement therapy. Lancet 1990;335:310–2.

48. Moorjani S, Dupont A, Labrie F, et al. Changes in plasma lipoprotein and apolipo-protein composition in relation to oral versus percutaneous administration alone or in cyclic association with utrogestan in menopausal women. J Clin Endocrinol Metab 1991;73:373–9.

49. Erpecum KJ, Van Berge Henegouwen GP, et al. Different hepatobiliary effects of oral and transdermal estradiol in postmenopausal women. Gastroenterology 1991;100:482–8.

50. Fitzpatrick LA, Pace C, Wiita B. Comparison of regimens containing oral micronized progesterone of medroxyprogesterone acetate on quality of life in postmenopausal women: a cross-sectional survey. J Womens Health Gend Based Med 2000;9:381–7.

51. Cummings JA, Brizendine L. Comparison of physical and emotional side effects of progesterone or medroxyprogesterone in early postmenopausal women. Meno-pause 2002;9:253–63.

52. Lindenfeld EA, Langer RD. Bleeding patterns of the hormone replacement therapies in the postmenopausal estrogen and progestin interventions trial. Obstet Gynecol 2002;100(5 Pt 1):853–63.

53. Greendale GA, Reboussin BA, Hogan P, et al. Symptom relief and side effects of postmenopausal hormones: results from the Postmenopausal Estrogen/Progestin Interventions Trial. Obstet Gynecol 1998;92(6):982–8.

54. Hargrove JT, Maxson WS, Wentz AC, et al. Menopausal hormone replacement therapy with continuous daily oral micronized progesterone. Obstet Gynecol 1989;73:606–12.

55. Holtorf K. The bioidentical hormone debate: Are bioidentical hormones (estradiol, estriol, and progesterone) safer or more efficacious than commonly used synthetic versions in hormone replacement therapy? Postgrad Med 2009;121:73–85.

56. Wood CE, Register TC, Lees CJ, et al. Effects of estradiol with micronized proges-terone or medroxyprogesterone acetate on risk markers for breast cancer in post-menopausal monkeys. Breast Cancer Res Treat 2007;101:125–34.

57. Inoh A, Kamiya K, Fujii Y, et al. Protective effects of progesterone and tamoxifen in estrogen induced mammary carcinogenesis in ovariectomized W/Fu rats. Jpn J Cancer Res 1985;76:699–704.

58. Malet C, Spritzer P, Guillaumin D, et al. Progesterone effect on cell growth, ultra-structural aspect and estradiol receptors of normal breast epithelial (HBE) cells in culture. J Steroid Biochem Mol Biol 2000;73:171–81.

59. Soderqvist G, von Schoultz B, Tani E, et al. Estrogen and progesterone receptor content in breast epithelial cells from healthy women during the menstrual cycle. Am J Obstet Gynecol 1993;168(3 Pt 1):874–9.

60. Formby B, Wiley TS. Progesterone inhibits growth and induces apoptosis in breast cancer cells: inverse effects on Bcl-2 and p53. Ann Clin Lab Sci 1998;28:360–9.

61. Warren MP. A comparative review of the risks and benefits of hormone replacement therapy regimens. Am J Obstet Gynecol 2004;190:1141–67.

62. de Lignières B. Effects of progestogens on the postmenopausal breast. Climacteric 2002;5:229–35.

63. Campagnoli C, Clavel-Chapelon F, Kaaks R, et al. Progestins and progesterone in hormone replacement therapy and the risk of breast cancer. J Steroid Biochem Mol Biol 2005;96:95–108.

64. Ory K, Lebeau J, Levalois C, et al. Apoptosis inhibition mediated by medroxypro-gesterone acetate treatment of breast cancer cell lines. Breast Cancer Res Treat 2001;68:187–98.

101. Collaborative Group on Hormonal Factors in Breast Cancer. Breast cancer and hormone replacement therapy: collaborative reanalysis of data from 51 epidemiological studies of 52,705 women with breast cancer and 108,411 women without breast cancer. Lancet 1997;350:1047–59.

102. Schairer C, Lubin J, Troisi R, et al. Menopausal estrogen and estrogen-progestin replacement therapy and breast cancer risk. JAMA 2000;283:485–91.

103. Colditz G, Rosner B. Use of estrogen plus progestin is associated with greater increase in breast cancer risk than estrogen alone. Am J Epidemiol 1998;147:S45.

104. Persson I, Weiderpass E, Bergkvist L, et al. Risks of breast and endometrial cancer after estrogen and estrogen-progestin replacement. Cancer Causes Control 1999; 10:253–60.

105. Chen CL, Weiss NS, Newcomb P, et al. Hormone replacement therapy in relation to breast cancer. JAMA 2002;287:734–41.

106. Pike MC, Ross RK. Progestins and menopause: epidemiological studies of risks of endometrial and breast cancer. Steroids 2000;65:659–64.

107. Santen RJ, Pinkerton J, McCartney C, et al. Risk of breast cancer with progestins in combination with estrogen as hormone replacement therapy. J Clin Endocrinol Metab 2001;86:16–23.

108. Stahlberg C, Pederson AT, Lynge E, et al. Hormone replacement therapy and risk of breast cancer: the role of progestins. Acta Obstet Gynecol Scand 2003;82:335–44.

109. Olsson HL, Ingvar C, Bladström A. Hormone replacement therapy containing progestins and given continuously increases breast carcinoma risk in Sweden. Cancer 2003;97:1387–92.

110. Colditz GA, Hankinson SE, Hunter DJ, et al. The use of estrogens and progestins and the risk of breast cancer in postmenopausal women. N Engl J Med 1995;332: 1589–93.

111. Colditz GA, Rosner B. Cumulative risk of breast cancer to age 70 years according to risk factor status: data from the Nurses' Health Study. Am J Epidemiol 2000;152: 950–64.

112. Peck JD, Hulka BS, Poole C, et al. Steroid hormone levels during pregnancy and incidence of maternal breast cancer. Cancer Epidemiol Biomarkers Prev 2002;11: 361–8.

113. Micheli A, Muti P, Secreto G, et al. Endogenous sex hormones and subsequent breast cancer in premenopausal women. Int J Cancer 2004;112:312–8.

114. Bernstein L, Yuan JM, Ross RK, et al. Serum hormone levels in pre-menopausal Chinese women in Shanghai and white women in Los Angeles: results from two breast cancer case-control studies. Cancer Causes Control 1990;1:51–8.

115. Drafta D, Schindler AE, Milcu SM, et al. Plasma hormones in pre- and postmenopausal breast cancer. J Steroid Biochem 1980;13:793–802.

116. Malarkey WB, Schroeder LL, Stevens VC, et al. Twenty-four-hour preoperative endocrine profiles in women with benign and malignant breast disease. Cancer Res 1977;37:4655–9.

117. Meyer F, Brown JB, Morrison AS, et al. Endogenous sex hormones, prolactin, and breast cancer in premenopausal women. J Natl Cancer Inst 1986;77:613–6.

118. Secreto G, Toniolo P, Berrino F, et al. Increased androgenic activity and breast cancer risk in premenopausal women. Cancer Res 1984(12 Pt 1);44:5902–5.

119. Cowan LD, Gordis L, Tonascia JA, et al. Breast cancer incidence in women with a history of progesterone deficiency. Am J Epidemiol 1981;114:209–17.

120. Badwe RA, Wang DY, Gregory WM, et al. Serum progesterone at the time of surgery and survival in women with premenopausal operable breast cancer. Eur J Cancer 1994;30A:445–8.

121. Mohr PE, Wang DY, Gregory WM, et al. Serum progesterone and prognosis in operable breast cancer. Br J Cancer 1996;73:1552–5.
122. DeLignieres B, de Vathaire F, Fournier S, et al. Combined hormone replacement therapy and risk of breast cancer in a French cohort study of 3175 women. Climacteric 2002;5:332–40.
123. Bakken K, Alsaker E, Eggen AE, et al. Hormone replacement therapy and incidence of hormone-dependent cancers in the Norwegian Women and Cancer study. Int J Cancer 2004;112:130–4.
124. Ottosson UB, Johansson BG, von Schoultz B. Subfractions of high-density lipoprotein cholesterol during estrogen replacement therapy: a comparison between progestogens and natural progesterone. Am J Obstet Gynecol 1985;151:746–50.
125. Minshall RD, Stanczyk FZ, Miyagawa K, et al. Ovarian steroid protection against coronary artery hyperreactivity in rhesus monkeys. J Clin Endocrinol Metab 1998; 83:649–59.
126. Mishra RG, Hermsmeyer RK, Miyagawas K, et al. Medroxyprogesterone acetate and dihydrotestosterone induce coronary hyperreactivity in intact male rhesus monkeys. J Clin Endocrinol Metab 2005;90:3706–14.
127. Miyagawa K, Roöch J, Stanczyk F, et al. Medroxyprogesterone interferes with ovarian steroid protection against coronary vasospasm. Nat Med 1997;3:324–7.
128. Saarikoski S, Yliskoski M, Penttilä I. Sequential use of norethisterone and natural progesterone in pre-menopausal bleeding disorders. Maturitas 1990;12:89–97.
129. Ottosson UB. Oral progesterone and estrogen/progestogen therapy. Effects of natural and synthetic hormones on subfractions of HDL cholesterol and liver proteins. Acta Obstet Gynecol Scand Suppl 1984;127:1–37.
130. Rosano GM, Webb CM, Chierchia S, et al. Natural progesterone, but not medroxyprogesterone acetate, enhances the beneficial effect of estrogen on exercise-induced myocardial ischemia in postmenopausal women. J Am Coll Cardiol 2000; 36:2154–9.
131. Otsuki M, Saito H, Xu X, et al. Progesterone, but not medroxyprogesterone, inhibits vascular cell adhesion molecule-1 expression in human vascular endothelial cells. Arterioscler Thromb Vasc Biol 2001;21:243–8.
132. Wagner JD, Martino MA, Jayo MJ, et.al. The effects of hormone replacement therapy on carbohydrate metabolism and cardiovascular risk factors in surgically postmenopausal cynomolgus monkeys. Metabolism 1996;45:1254–62.
133. Jensen J, Riis BJ, Strøm V, et al. Long-term effects of percutaneous estrogens and oral progesterone on serum lipoproteins in postmenopausal women. Am J Obstet Gynecol 1987;156:66–71.
134. Williams JK, Honoré EK, Washburn SA, et al. Effects of hormone replacement on therapy on reactivity of atherosclerotic coronary arteries in cynomolgus monkeys. J Am Coll Cardiol 1994;24:1757–61.
135. Adams MR, Kaplan JR, Manuck SB, et al. Inhibition of coronary artery atherosclerosis by 17-beta estradiol in ovariectomized monkeys. Arteriosclerosis 1990;10: 1051–7.
136. Bolaji II, Grimes H, Mortimer G, et al. Low-dose progesterone therapy in oestrogenised postmenopausal women: effects on plasma lipids, lipoproteins and liver function parameters. Eur J Obstet Gynecol Reprod Biol 1993;48:61–8.
137. Morey AK, Pedram A, Razandi M, et al. Estrogen and progesterone inhibit vascular smooth muscle proliferation. Endocrinology 1997;138:3330–9.
138. Lee WS, Harder JA, Yoshizumi M, et al. Progesterone inhibits arterial smooth muscle cell proliferation. Nat Med 1997;3:1005–8.

139. Jeanes HL, Wanikiat P, Sharif I, et al. Medroxyprogesterone acetate inhibits the cardioprotective effect of estrogen in experimental ischemia-reperfusion injury. Menopause 2006;13:80–6.

140. Hirvonen E, Malkonen M, Manninen V. Effects of different progestogens on lipoproteins during postmenopausal replacement therapy. N Engl J Med 1981;304:560–3.

141. Feeman WE Jr. Thrombotic stroke in an otherwise healthy middle-aged female related to the use of continuous-combined conjugated equine estrogens and medroxyprogesterone acetate. J Gend Specif Med 2000;3:62–4.

142. Lindheim SR, Presser SC, Ditkoff EC, et al. A possible bimodal effect of estrogen on insulin sensitivity in postmenopausal women and the attenuating effect of added progestin. Fertil Steril 1993;60:664–7.

143. Spencer CP, Godsland IF, Cooper AJ, et al. Effects of oral and transdermal 17β-estradiol with cyclical oral norethindrone acetate on insulin sensitivity, secretion, and elimination in postmenopausal women. Metabolism 2000;49:742–7.

144. Godsland IF, Gangar K, Walton C,et al. Insulin resistance, secretion, and elimination in postmenopausal women receiving oral or transdermal hormone replacement therapy. Metabolism1993;42:846–53.

145. Adams MR, Register TC, Golden DL, et al. Medroxyprogesterone acetate antagonizes inhibitory effects of conjugated equine estrogens on coronary artery atherosclerosis. Arterioscler Thromb Vasc Biol 1997;17:217–21.

146. Levine RL, Chen SJ, Durand J, et al. Medroxyprogesterone attenuates estrogen-mediated inhibition of neointima formation after balloon injury of the rat carotid artery. Circulation 1996;94:2221–7.

147. Register TC, Adams MR, Golden DL, et al. Conjugated equine estrogens alone, but not in combination with medroxyprogesterone acetate, inhibit aortic connective tissue remodeling after plasma lipid lowering in female monkeys. Arterioscler Thromb Vasc Biol 1998;18:1164–71.

148. Fåhraeus L, Larsson-Cohn U, Wallentin L. L-Norgestrel and progesterone have different influences on plasma lipoproteins. Eur J Clin Invest 1983;13:447–53.

149. The Women's Health Initiative Participant Website. Effects of estrogen-alone on stroke in the Women's Health Initiative. Findings summary. Available at: http://www.whi.org/findings/ht/ealone_stroke.php. Accessed March 17, 2011.

150. Zumoff B, Strain Gw, Miller LK, et al. Twenty-four-hour mean plasma testosterone concentration declines with age in normal premenopausal women. J Clin Endorinol Metab 1995;80:1429–30.

151. Braunstein GD. Androgen insufficiency in women: a summary of critical issues. Fertil Steril 2002;77:S94–S99.

152. Miller KK, Rosner W. Lee H, et al. Measurement of free testosterone in normal women and women with androgen deficiency: Comparison of methods. J Clin Endocrinol Metab 2004;89:525–33.

153. Rosner W, Auchus RJ, Azziz R, et al. Position statement: utility, limitations, and pitfalls in measuring testosterone: an endocrine society position statement. J Clin Endocrinol Metab 2007;92:405–13.

154. Gelst SH. Androgen therapy in gynecology. JAMA 1940;117:2207–13.

155. Sherwin BB, Gelfand MM, Brender W. Androgen enhances sexual motivation in females: a prospective, crossover study of sex steroid administration in the surgical menopause. Psychosom Med 1985;47:339–51.

156. Burger H, Hailes J, Nelson J, et al. Effect of combined implants of estradiol and testosterone on libido in postmenopausal women. Br Med J (Clin Res Ed) 1987;294:936–7.

157. Davis SR, McCloud P, Strauss BJG, et al. Testosterone enhances estradiol's effect on postmenopausal bone density and sexuality. Maturitas 1995;21:227–36.
158. Floter A, Nathorst-Boos J, Carlstrom K, et al. Addition of testosterone to estrogen replacement therapy in oophorectomized women: effects on sexuality and well-being. Climacteric 2002;5:357–65.
159. Shifren JL, Braunstein GD, Simon JA, et al. Transdermal testosterone treatment in women with impaired sexual function after oophorectomy. N Engl J Med 2000;343: 682–8.
160. Montgomery JC, Appleby L, Brincat M, et al. Effect of oestrogen and testosterone implants on psychological disorders in the climacteric. Lancet 1987;1:297–9.
161. Sherwin BB. Affective changes with estrogen and androgen replacement therapy in surgically menopausal women. J Affect Disord 1988;14:177–87.
162. Sherwin BB, Gelfand M. Differential symptom response to parenteral estrogen and/or androgen administration in the surgical menopause. Am J Obstet Gynecol 1985;151:153–60.
163. Davis S, Walker K. Effects of estradiol with and without testosterone on body composition and relationship with lipids in postmenopausal women. Menopause 2000;7:395–401.
164. Dobs A, Nguyen T. Differential effects of oral estrogen versus oral estrogen-androgen replacement therapy on body composition in postmenopausal women. Clin Endocrinol Metab 2002;87:1509–16.
165. Watts NB, Notelovitz M, Timmons MC, et al. Comparison of oral estrogens and estrogen plus androgen on bone mineral density, menopausal symptoms and lipid-lipoprotein profiles in surgical menopause. Obstet Gynecol 1995;85:529–37.
166. Slemenda C, Longcope C, Peacock M, et al. Sex steroids, bone mass, and bone loss. A prospective study of pre-, peri- and postmenopausal women. J Clin Invest 1996;97:14–21.
167. Braunstein GD, Sundwall DA, Katz M, et al. Safety and efficacy of a testosterone patch for the treatment of hypoactive sexual desire disorder in surgically menopausal women: a randomized, placebo-controlled trial. Arch Intern Med 2005;165:1582–9.
168. Simon J, Braunstein G, Nachtigall L, et al. Testosterone patch increases sexual activity and desire in surgically menopausal women with hypoactive sexual desire disorder: results of the Intimate SM 1 study. J Clin Endocrinol Metab 2005;90: 5226–33.
169. Buckler HM, McElhone K, Durrington PN, et al. The effects of low-dose testosterone treatment on lipid metabolism, clotting factors and ultrasonographic ovarian morphology in women. Clin Endocrinol 1998;49:173–8.
170. Floter A, Nathorst-Boos J, Carlstrom K, et al. Serum lipids in oophorectomized women during estrogen and testosterone replacement therapy. Maturitas 2004;47:123–9.
171. Dimitrakakis C, Jones RA, Lin A, et al. Breast cancer incidence in postmenopausal women using testosterone in addition to usual hormone therapy. Menopause 2004;11:531–5.
172. Hubayter A, Simon JA. Testosterone therapy for sexual dysfunction in postmenopausal women. Climateric 2008;11:181–91.
173. Goldstat R, Briganti E, Tran J, et al. Transdermal testosterone therapy improves well-being, mood, and sexual function in premenopausal women. Menopause 2003;10:390–8.
174. Tuiten A, Van Honk J, Koppeschaar H, et al. Time course of effects of testosterone administration on sexual arousal in women. Arch Gen Psychiatry 2000;57:149–53.

Hormone Replacement Therapy in the Geriatric Patient: Current State of the Evidence and Questions for the Future—Estrogen, Progesterone, Testosterone, and Thyroid Hormone Augmentation in Geriatric Clinical Practice: Part 2

Erika Schwartz, MD[a],*, Vincent Morelli, MD[b], Kent Holtorf, MD[c]

KEYWORDS
- Hormone replacement therapy • Testosterone • Elderly
- Thyroid hormone • Frailty • T_3 • T_4 • Hypothyroidism

TESTOSTERONE

The first modern description of the effects of testosterone on men was by Dr Charles Brown-Sequard, in 1889 when, upon self-injection of testicular extracts from different animals, he reported increased energy, muscular strength, stamina, and mental agility.[1] Since that time, hundreds of studies have described testosterone's physiologic effects, the declining testosterone levels that occur normally with aging and the physiologic and psychological effects of replacement therapy.

Physiologic Effects

Testosterone's physiologic effects are well documented[2–5] and include increasing muscle mass, increasing hepatic synthesis of clotting factors, altering other hepatic enzymes, decreasing HDL, increasing bone mineral density, and increasing erythropoietin

The authors have nothing to disclose.
[a] Age Management Institute, 200 West 57 Street, Suite 502, New York, NY 10019, USA
[b] Department of Family and Community Medicine, Meharry Medical College, 1005 Dr D.B. Todd, Jr, Boulevard, Nashville, TN, USA
[c] Holtorf Medical Group, Torrance, CA, USA
* Corresponding author.
E-mail address: Eschwartz@ageMD.org

Clin Geriatr Med 27 (2011) 561–575
doi:10.1016/j.cger.2011.07.004
0749-0690/11/$ – see front matter © 2011 Elsevier Inc. All rights reserved.

geriatric.theclinics.com

synthesis. These effects lead to potential benefits as well as risks associated with testosterone supplementation.

Normal Decline With Aging

Testosterone levels decline 1% to 1.5% per year after age 30,[6] and the prevalence of low testosterone (total testosterone <300 ng/dL) is as high as 38.7% in males over the age of 45 in outpatient primary care populations.[7]

Effects of Low Serum Testosterone

The normal age-related decline in testosterone levels (andropause) has been associated with, and is often thought to contribute to, a number of "age-related symptoms." These symptoms include muscle loss (sarcopenia), depression, decreased strength and physical performance, decreased bone density, central obesity, insulin resistance, loss of libido, and erectile dysfunction.[8] Low serum testosterone has also been associated with obesity, dyslipidemias,[9] type 2 diabetes,[10–12] and the metabolic syndrome.[13]

In addition, age-related declines in testosterone have been associated with an increased all cause mortality in aging men. A 2006 study[14] followed 858 participants for an average of 4.3 years and found that low serum testosterone was associated with higher all-cause mortality. The results of this study were reinforced in 2007 when Khaw and colleagues[15] followed 11,606 men (ages 40–70) for 10 years and again found that low endogenous testosterone levels were associated with significantly greater all-cause mortality, cardiovascular-related mortality, and cancer-related mortality. Men in the highest quartile testosterone levels were found to have 30% reduction in mortality compared with those in the lowest quartile.[15]

DEFINITION OF HYPOGONADISM IN OLDER MEN

There is no agreed upon definition of hypogonadism in older men, and most physicians use a combination of clinical signs and serum testosterone measurements to determine whether hypogonadism exists and whether or not testosterone replacement therapy may be indicated.[16,17] Some investigators use a total testosterone level of 200 ng/dL as a cutoff value for hypogonadism regardless of age,[18,19] whereas others consider individuals whose total testosterone levels of less than 300 ng/dL to be hypogonadal.[20,21]

Total serum testosterone is the most commonly used measurement of androgen activity, although it is a poor indicator of tissue activity[22,23] and demonstrates little correlation with clinical status.[24] In addition, total testosterone levels are unreliable indicators of response to therapy.[17,25] Free testosterone measurements are equally inaccurate in the clinical setting,[23] with normal ranges varying widely between laboratories and bearing little correlation to clinical findings.[22] Bioavailable testosterone measures the total free and loosely bound testosterone. Free and bioavailable testosterone levels are potentially better markers of active testosterone levels, but are presently not clinically useful.

It also may be simplistic to think solely in terms of serum levels as indicators of tissue androgen activity, and it must also be remembered that counterbalancing hormone states (ie, cortisol, estrogen acting as anti-androgens), androgen receptor status, and gene expression may also play roles in androgen activity. Although total serum measurements are suboptimal, clinicians are usually left using this measurement in their evaluation of hypogonadism. It is important that they keep in mind the limitations of this metric.

As background, it must be remembered that greater than 95% of total testosterone in the blood is either tightly bound to sex hormone-binding globulin (SHBG) or loosely bound to albumin and other serum proteins, leaving less than 5% unbound as free testosterone. Testosterone bound to SHBG is inactive because it is unavailable to enter the cells, whereas albumin-bound testosterone can separate from its carrier protein and become free, and thus useful, at the cellular level. Higher SHBG levels mean more bound and less free testosterone, whereas lower SHBG levels indicate the opposite. However, the clinical usefulness of taking the SHBG into consideration when evaluating testosterone levels remains elusive, and most authors use total serum testosterone measurements in their evaluations of hypogonadism.

In addition, it must be remembered that when testing a symptomatic elderly patients it is unusual to have prior (younger) testosterone levels available for comparison. Thus, a level that is within the normal range may reflect a significant decline from an individual's "younger baseline" level, and thus may be "low" for that individual patient. The lack of optimal serum testosterone measurements and this individual variation of normal is why many authors emphasize the importance of clinical assessment in evaluating for hypogonadism.

EFFECTS OF TESTOSTERONE SUPPLEMENTATION

Over the last 30 years, many small, short-term studies have pointed to several beneficial effects of testosterone supplementation.

Cardiovascular Benefits

Small studies show that the administration of exogenous testosterone improves myocardial perfusion, increases exercise time in patients with cardiovascular disease and lowers testosterone levels.[26–28] However, there exists more potential cardiovascular risks than benefits with supplementation.

Frailty

Although there is no universally accepted definition of frailty, one can get a general sense of it by considering 2 of the commonly used characterizations. The first is, "Frailty is a clinical syndrome characterized by reduced physiologic reserve affecting multiple organ systems and is associated with increased risk of falls, fractures, hospitalization and death." A second definition of frailty, set out in 2001 by a John Hopkins University Study, defines frailty as, "A clinical syndrome in which three or more of the following criteria are present: unintentional weight loss (the pounds in the past year), self-reported exhaustion, weakness, slow walking speed, and low physical activity."[29] Despite the lack of standard definition, frailty is generally agreed to be a "pre-disability state" with characteristics of anorexia, sarcopenia, immobility, balance deficits, depression and cognitive impairment"[30]—all conditions seemingly ripe for intervention with testosterone replacement therapy.

In a 2010 randomized trial of 99 hypogonadal elderly men (age >60, total testosterone <350), with frailty (≥1 of the Hopkins criteria mentioned above) and a bone density T-score less than −2, participants were randomized to receive either 5 mg of AndroGel or placebo daily. At the end of the 12- to 24-month study period, testosterone supplementation was shown to increase skeletal and lean body mass; to increase axial bone density; but have no significant effect on femur bone density, muscle strength, or physical performance. There were no differences in side effects between groups.[31]

In another study, the largest randomized testosterone replacement trial in elderly men to date (published in 2010),[32] 274 hypogonadal men (total testosterone < 350 with at least 1 of the 5 above frailty characteristics) were randomized to receive either placebo or transdermal testosterone and followed for 6 months. Lower extremity muscle strength (but not grip strength) was significantly improved in the treatment group. However, it should also be noted that most previous interventional studies[33-38] were unable to demonstrate improvements in lower limb strength. Lean body mass was significantly improved in the treatment arm in this and several other studies. Physical function was not significantly improved in this study either. However, when subgroup analysis was considered there was significant improvement in some physical performance tests among older men who exhibited a greater degree of frailty. Quality-of-life improvements were noted by the Aging Male Syndrome questionnaire in somatic and sexual functioning but not in psychological symptoms.

The latest study assessing muscular function and strength in elderly hypogonadal men was published in 2010 in the *New England Journal of Medicine*.[39] This study of 209 men demonstrated increased leg press strength, chest press strength, and loaded stair climbing.

In summary, testosterone supplementation in frail hypogonadal men will produce an increase in lean body mass, and may provide a modest benefit in muscle strength and physical performance, especially in the frailest subgroups. It also may provide subjective improvement in somatic and sexual functioning. There is no demonstrated benefit in fall prevention. Not a very strong endorsement for testosterone's use in frail hypogonadal men.

Depression

Early observational studies noted lower bioavailable serum testosterone levels in depressed men[40] providing the rational for investigating the effects of testosterone replacement therapy in depressed older men. Several studies have been done with conflicting results.

A 2009 systemic meta-analysis by Zarrouf and colleagues[41] evaluated 7 placebo-controlled, randomized trials (n = 364) comparing testosterone replacement with placebo in depressed men. Overall results revealed a significant positive response to testosterone therapy in hypogonadal patients.

However, the 2 most recent studies revealed no significant effect of testosterone replacement on depressed hypogonadal elderly men.[32,42] The latter study, published in 2010 out of Harvard University, failed to show any benefit from testosterone gel supplementation in depressed hypogonadal (serum testosterone <350 ng/dL) men who were resistant to selective serotonin reuptake inhibitor treatment. The authors concluded that, "The possibility remains that testosterone might benefit a particular subgroup of depressed men, but if so, the characteristics of this subgroup would still need to be established."

Cognitive Function

Although higher serum testosterone levels have associated with improved cognition[43] and some short-term augmentation trials have demonstrated improvements in verbal and spatial memory,[44] longer trials have been conflicting, less optimistic and have demonstrated little or no change in cognitive functioning.[45,46]

Sexual Function

The effect of testosterone replacement therapy on sexual function in hypogonadal men is not clear. Recent studies and meta-analyses have conflicting results. A 2005 meta-analysis[47] of 17 randomized trials (n = 656), concluded that hypogonadal men (serum testosterone <12 pg/mL or <350 ng/dL), experienced moderate improvement in number of nocturnal erections, sexual thoughts, successful intercourse, and sexual satisfaction with testosterone replacement therapy. (No such effects were documented in eugonadal men.) The authors go on to say, however, that their results must be viewed with caution as the quality of studies included were suboptimal—being small, of short duration, with considerable heterogeneity, and subject to publication bias and reporting data "without proper statistical considerations." They note that a large-scale, prospective trial in hypogonadal men should be performed to definitively elucidate testosterone replacement's role in sexual function.

A more recent meta-analysis published in *Mayo Clinic Proceedings* in 2007[48] evaluated 17 studies with 862 participants and concluded that *hypogonadal men* showed a significant improvement in libido, a nonsignificant improvement with satisfaction of erectile function, and no significant effect on sexual satisfaction. In men with normal serum testosterone levels, results showed a small effect on erectile function but no significant effects on libido or overall sexual function.

Finally, the latest randomized trial of testosterone replacement therapy in hypogonadal men was published in 2009.[49] This 6-month trial involving 207 participants revealed no change in sexual fantasies, sexual desire, or frequency of sexual contact in the treatment arm.

At this point, one must conclude that testosterone replacement may, at best, modestly improve some but not all aspects of sexual functioning.

POTENTIAL SIDE EFFECTS

The untoward effects of *supraphysiologic* doses of testosterone are well known and well documented and include weight gain, sleep apnea, gynecomastia, acne, increased hematocrit (from increased synthesis of clotting factors), hypercoagulable syndromes (strokes[50] and heart attacks have been reported[51]), hemorrhagic liver cysts, liver failure, and liver cancer (usually only with alkylated androgens).

The most concerning side effects of physiologic replacement (testosterone supplementation to bring serum levels back to normal) to date comes from a Boston University study published in the *New England Journal of Medicine* in 2010.[39] In this study, 176 hypogonadal men with a high degree of comorbidities (eg, diabetes, cardiovascular disease, hyperlipidemia) were randomized to receive either transdermal testosterone or placebo for 6 months. The study was meant to assess strength gains with testosterone supplementation but was terminated early owing to an increase in cardiovascular events in the testosterone group. (Cardiac events included myocardial infarction, acute coronary syndrome, congestive heart failure exacerbation, and rising blood pressure; 23 untoward cardiac events in the treatment arm vs 5 in the placebo group.)

In addition, concerns about the development of benign prostate hyperplasia while on testosterone replacement exist. In the few studies addressing this issue, prostate volumes have indeed been reported to modestly increase with testosterone replacement therapy; however, this increase has only returned the prostate to a "eugonadal size" (normal-sized prostate for a man with normal serum testosterone levels). In addition, patients in the 1-year studies cited below did not experience any increase in obstructive symptoms.[52,53] The most recent study (1998) examining the question of prostate size and supplementation found no increase in prostate size after 15 weeks of testosterone supplementation in 31 healthy males.[54]

Concerns about prostate cancer with testosterone administration have been present for greater than 60 years.[55] However, an extensive review of the literature published out of Harvard in 2007 failed to establish a connection between high serum

As a result, when relying on serum tests only, clinicians do not treat patients presenting with this thyroid picture assuming they are euthyroid (normal T3, low T4, and normal TSH). Unfortunately, this situation limits our understanding of the physiologic changes occurring at the cellular level leaving a gaping hole and missing the opportunity to help the patients' condition.[83,84]

Aging and chronic illness also affect the hypothalamic–pituitary–thyroid–cellular axis. Both states tend to present with decreased TSH, decreased conversion of T4 to T3 in the cell, and increased reverse *T3* levels.[84,85] In these cases, serum reverse T3 levels may be a useful indicator of low tissue T3 levels because diminished cellular

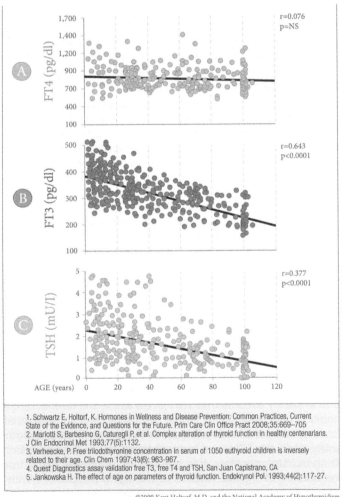

1. Schwartz E, Holtorf, K. Hormones in Wellness and Disease Prevention: Common Practices, Current State of the Evidence, and Questions for the Future. Prim Care Clin Office Pract 2008;35:669–705
2. Mariotti S, Barbesino G, Caturegli P, et al. Complex alteration of thyroid function in healthy centenarians. J Clin Endocrinol Met 1993;77(5):1132.
3. Verheecke, P. Free triiodothyronine concentration in serum of 1050 euthyroid children is inversely related to their age. Clin Chem 1997;43(6): 963-967.
4. Quest Diagnostics assay validation free T3, free T4 and TSH, San Juan Capistrano, CA
5. Jankowska H. The effect of age on parameters of thyroid function. Endokrynol Pol. 1993;44(2):117-27.

©2009 Kent Holtorf, M.D. and the National Academy of Hypothyroidism

Fig. 1. Age dependent variations in mean serum levels of Free T4 (A), Free T3 (B) and TSH (C) in healthy individuals-a combined analysis of the literature. Demonstrates that TSH is not a reliable marker of active thyroid (T3) levels (low T3 levels are associated with decreased, not increased, TSH levels). (*Courtesy of* Kent Holtorf, MD and the National Academy of Hypothyroidism.)

uptake of T4, diminished T4 to T3 conversion and diminished cellular T3 levels correlate inversely with serum reverse T3 levels.[85]

Another finding in the aging patient is a reduction in TSH response to thyrotropin-releasing hormone from the pituitary, resulting in depressed levels of TSH. This suppression is similar to the TSH suppression found in severely ill patients with documented nonthyroidal illness (**Fig. 1**).[94,96] TSH failure to respond to thyrotropin-releasing hormone stimulation in the elderly further contributes to confusing information gained from standard thyroid testing in this population. Increased incidence of systemic illness and multiple medications in the elderly also directly affect thyroid function, further reducing the accuracy of the standard thyroid tests (T4 and TSH) as markers of true thyroid status.

In aging patients who present with symptoms consistent with hypothyroidism but have a normal TSH and T4 level, a T3/rT3 ratio may help gain more insight of tissue thyroid status. Optimal tissue levels are associated with a free T3/rT3 ratio greater than 1.8. (free T3 is reported in picograms per deciliter and reverse T3 in picograms per deciliter).[81–93]

Although there are limitations in all type of testing for this age group, obtaining free tri-iodothyronine, reverse tri-iodothyronine, and tri-iodothyronine/reverse tri-iodothyronine ratios may be helpful to provide a somewhat accurate evaluation of tissue thyroid status and may predict favorable responders to thyroid supplementation.

Treatment

Thyroid replacement is not reported as beneficial during acute stress. When the stress is chronic or age-related treatment with T3 (liothyronine [Cytomel; Jones Pharma,

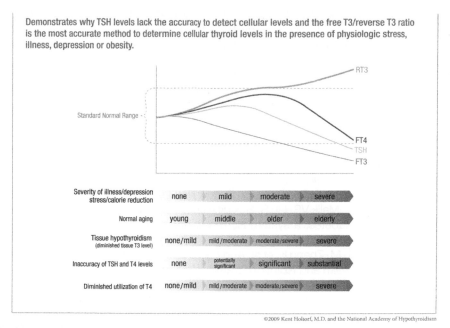

©2009 Kent Holtorf, M.D. and the National Academy of Hypothyroidism

Fig. 2. Associated serum thyroid levels with progressively decreasing tissue thyroid levels due to stress, illness, depression, calorie reduction or aging (Why standard blood tests lack sensitivity to detect low thyroid in the presence of such conditions). (*Courtesy of* Kent Holtorf, MD and the National Academy of Hypothyroidism.)

35. Clague JE, Wu FC, Horan MA. Difficulties in measuring the effect of testosterone replacement therapy on muscle function in older men. Int J Androl 1999;22:261–5.

36. Wittert GA, Chapman IM, Haren MT, et al. Oral testosterone supplementation increases muscle and decreases fat mass in healthy elderly males with low-normal gonadal status. J Gerontol A Biol Sci Med Sci 2003;58:618–625.

37. Brill KT, Weltman AL, Gentili A, et al. Single and combined effects of growth hormone and testosterone administration on measures of body composition, physical performance, mood, sexual function, bone turnover, and muscle gene expression in healthy older men. J Clin Endocrinol Metab 2002;87:5649–57.

38. Nair KS, Rizza RA, O'Brien P, et al. DHEA in elderly women and DHEA or testosterone in elderly men. N Engl J Med 2006;355:1647–59.

39. Basaria S, Coviello AD, Travison TG, et al. Adverse events associated with testosterone administration. N Engl J Med 2010;363:109–22.

40. Barrett-Conner E, Von Muhlen DG, Kritz-Silverstein D. Bioavailable testosterone and depressed mood in older men: the Rancho Bernardo Study. J Clin Endocrinol Metab 1999;84:573–7.

41. Zarrouf FA, Artz S, Griffith J, et al. Testosterone and depression: systematic review and meta-analysis. J Psychiatr Pract 2009;15:289–305.

42. Pope HG Jr, Amiaz R, Brennan BP, et al. Parallel-group placebo-controlled trial of testosterone gel in men with major depressive disorder displaying an incomplete response to standard antidepressant treatment. J Clin Psychopharmacol 2010;30: 126–34.

43. Barrett-Connor E, Goodman-Gruen D, Patay B. Endogenous sex hormones and cognitive function in older men. J Clin Endocrinol Metab 1999;84:3681–5.

44. Cherrier MM, Asthana S, Plymate S, et al. Testosterone supplementation improves spatial and verbal memory in healthy older men. Neurology 2001;57:80–8.

45. Haren MT, Wittert GA, Chapman IM, et al. Effects of oral testosterone undecenoate on visuospatial cognition, mood and quality of like in elderly men with low-normal gonadal status. Maturitas 2005;50:124–33.

46. Emmelot-Vonk MH, Verhaar HJ, Nakhai Pour HR, et al. Effect of testosterone supplementation on functional mobility, cognition, and other parameters in older men: a randomized controlled trial. JAMA 2008;299:39–52.

47. Isidori AM, Giannetta E, Gianfrilli D, et al. Effects of testosterone on sexual function in men: results of a meta-analysis. Clin Endocrinol (Oxf) 2005;63:381–94.

48. Boloña ER, Uraga MV, Haddad RM, et al. Testosterone use in men with sexual dysfunction: a systematic review and meta-analysis of randomized placebo-controlled trials. Mayo Clin Proc 2007;82:20–8.

49. Emmelot-Vonk MH, Verhaar HJ, Nakhai-Pour HR, et al. Effect of testosterone supplementation on sexual functioning in aging men: a 6-month randomized controlled trial. Int J Impot Res 2009;21:129–38.

50. Frankle MA, Eichberg R, Zachariah SB. Anabolic androgenic steroids and a stroke in an athlete: case report. Arch Phys Med Rehab 1988;69:632–3.

51. McNutt RA, Ferenchick GS, Kirlin PC, et al. Acute myocardial infarction in a 22-year-old world class weight lifter using anabolic steroids. Am J Cardiol 1988;62: 164.

52. Meikle AW, Arver S, Dobs AS, et al. Prostate size in hypogonadal men treated with a nonscrotal permeation-enhanced testosterone transdermal system. Urology 1997;49:191–6.

53. Behre HM, Bohmeyer J, Nieschlag E. Prostate volume in testosterone-treated and untreated hypogonadal men in comparison to age-matched normal controls. Clin Endocrinol (Oxf) 1994;40:341–9.

54. Cooper CS, Perry PJ, Sparks AE, et al. Effect of exogenous testosterone on prostate volume, serum and semen prostate specific antigen levels in healthy young men. J Urol 1998;159:441–3.
55. Huggins C, Stevens RE Jr, Hodges CV. Studies on prostatic cancer II: the effects of castration on advanced carcinoma of the prostate gland. Arch Surg 1941;43: 209–23.
56. Morgentaler A. Testosterone replacement therapy and prostate cancer. Urol Clin North Am 2007;34:555–63.
57. Stattin P, Lumme S, Tenkanen L, et al. High levels of circulating testosterone are not associated with increased prostate cancer risk: a pooled prospective study. Int J Cancer 2004;108:418–24.
58. Barrett-Connor E, Garland C, McPhillips JB, et al. A prospective, population-based study of androstenedione, estrogens, and prostatic cancer. Cancer Res 1990;50: 169–73.
59. Parsons JK, Carter HB, Platz EA, et al. Serum testosterone and the risk of prostate cancer: potential implications for testosterone therapy. Cancer Epidemiol Biomarkers Prev 2005;14:2257–60.
60. Marks LS, Mazer NA, Mostaghel E, et al. Effect of testosterone replacement therapy on prostate tissue in men with late-onset hypogonadism: a randomized controlled trial. JAMA 2006;296:2351–61.
61. Bhasin S, Singh AB, Mac RP, et al. Managing the risks of prostate disease during testosterone replacement therapy in older men. J Androl 2003;24:299–311.
62. Liverman CT, Blazer DG. Testosterone and aging: clinical research directions. Institute of Medicine. Washington (DC): National Academies Press; 2004.
63. Canaris GJ, Manowitz NR, Mayor G, et al. The Colorado thyroid disease prevalence study. Arch Intern Med 2000;160:526–34.
64. Mariotti S, Barbesino G, Caturegli P, et al. Complex alterations of thyroid function in healthy centenarians. J Clin Endocrinol Metab 1993;77:1130–4.
65. Van den Beld AW, Visser TJ, Feelders RA, et al. Thyroid hormone concentrations, disease, physical function and mortality in elderly men. J Clin Endocrinol Metab 2005;90:6403–9.
66. Magri F, Fioravanti CM, Vignati G, et al. Thyroid function in old and very old healthy subjects. J Endocrinol Invest 2002;25:60–3.
67. McDermott MT, Ridgway C. Subclinical hypothyroidism is mild thyroid failure and should be treated. J Clin Endocrinol Met 2001;86:4585–90.
68. Monzani F, Caraccio N, Del Guerra P, et al. Neuromuscular symptoms and dysfunction in subclinical hypothyroid patients: beneficial effect of L-T4 replacement therapy. Clin Endocrinol 1999;51:237–42.
69. Joffe RT, Levitt AJ. Major depression and subclinical (grade 2) hypothyroidism. Psychoneuroendocrinology 1992;17:215–21.
70. Haggerty JJ Jr, Stern RA, Mason GA, et al. Subclinical hypothyroidism: a modifiable risk factor for depression? Am J Psychiatry 1993;150:508–10.
71. Baldini IM, Vita A, Maura MC, et al. 1997 Psychological and cognitive features in subclinical hypothyroidism. Prog Neurophsychopharmacol Biol Psychiatry 1997;21: 925–35.
72. Danese MD, Ladenson PW, Meinert CL, et al. Effect of thyroxine therapy on serum lipoproteins in patients with mild thyroid failure: a quantitative review of the literature. J Clin Endocrinol Metab 2000;85:2993–3001.
73. Monzani F, Caraccio N, Siciliano G, et al. Clinical and biochemical features of muscle dysfunction in subclinical hypothyroidism. J Clin Endocrinol Metab 1997;82:3315–8.

74. Forfar JC, Wathen CG, Todd WT, et al. Left ventricular performance in subclinical hypothyroidism. QJM 1985;57:857–65.
75. Foldes J, Istvanfy M, Halmagyi M, et al. Hypothyroidism and the heart. Examination of left ventricular function in subclinical hypothyroidism. Acta Med Hung 1987;44: 337–47.
76. Kahaly GJ. Cardiovascular and atherogenic aspects of subclinical hypothyroidism. Thyroid 2000;10:665–79.
77. Walsh JP, Bremner AP, Bulsara MK, et al. Subclinical thyroid dysfunction as a risk factor for cardiovascular disease. Arch Intern Med 2005;165:2467–72.
78. Monzani F, Del Guerra P, Caraccio N, et al. Subclinical hypothyroidism: neurobehavioral features and beneficial effect of l-thyroxine treatment. Clin Invest 1993;71: 367–71.
79. Ridgway EC, Cooper DS, Walker H, et al. Peripheral responses to thyroid hormone before and after L-thyroxine therapy in patients with subclinical hypothyroidism. J Clin Endocrinol Metab 1981;53:1238–42.
80. Nystrom E, Caidahl K, Fager G, et al. A double-blind cross-over 12-month study of L-thyroxine treatment of women with 'subclinical' hypothyroidism. Clin Endocrinol 1988;29:63–76.
81. Docter R, Krenning EP, de Jong M, et al. The sick euthyroid syndrome: changes in thyroid hormone serum parameters and hormone metabolism. Clin Endocrinol (Oxf) 1993;39:499–518.
82. Peeters RP, Wouters PJ, Kaptein E, et al. Reduced activation and increased inactivation of thyroid hormone in tissues of critically ill patients. J Clin Endocrinol Metab 2003;88:3202–11.
83. Iervasi G, Pinitore A, Landi P, et al. Low-T3 syndrome a strong prognostic predictor of death in patients with heart disease. Circulation 2003;107:708–13.
84. Peeters RP, Wouters PJ, van Toor H, et al. Serum 3,3',5'-triiodothyronine (rT3) and 3,5,3'-triiodothyronine/rT3 are prognostic markers in critically ill patients and are associated with postmortem tissue deiodinase activities. J Clin Endocrinol Metab 2005;90:4559–65.
85. Chopra IJ, Solomon DH, Hepner GW, et al. Misleadingly low free thyroxine index and usefulness of reverse triiodothyronine measurement in nonthyroidal illnesses. Ann Intern Med 1979;90:905–12.
86. Carrero JJ, Qureshi AR, Axelsson J, et al. Clinical and biochemical implications of low thyroid hormone levels (total and free forms) in euthyroid patients with chronic kidney disease. J Intern Med 2007;262:690–701.
87. Zoccali C, Tripepi G, Cutrupi S, et al. Low triiodothyronine: a new facet of inflammation in end-stage renal disease. J Am Soc Nephrol 2005;16:2789–95.
88. Pingitore A, Landi P, Taddei MC, et al. Triiodothyronine levels for risk stratification of patients with chronic heart failure. Am J Med 2005;118:132–6.
89. Kozdag G, Ural D, Vural A, et al. Relation between free triiodothyronine/free thyroxine ratio, echocardiographic parameters and mortality in dilated cardiomyopathy. Eur J Heart Fail 2005;7:113–8.
90. Pingitore A, Galli E, Barison A, et al. Acute effects of triiodothyronine replacement therapy in patients with chronic heart failure and low T3 syndrome: a randomized placebo-controlled study. J Clin Endocrinol Met 2008;93:1351–8.
91. Dulchavsky SA, Kennedy PR, Geller ER, et al. T3 preserves respiratory function in sepsis. J Trauma 1991;31:753–9.
92. Meyer T, Husch M, van den Berg E, et al. Treatment of dopamine-dependent shock with triiodothyronine: preliminary results. Deutsch Med Wochenschr 1979;104: 1711–4.

93. Hamilton MA, Stevenson LW, Fonarow GC, et al. Safety and hemodynamic effects of intravenous triiodothyronine in advanced congestive heart failure. Am J Cardiol 1998;81:443–7.

94. Van Coevorden A, Laurent E, Decoster C, et al. Decreased basal and stimulated thyrotropin secretion in healthy elderly men. J Clin Endocrinol Metab 1989;69: 177–85.

95. Hermann J, Heinen E, Kroll HJ, et al. Thyroid function and thyroid hormone metabolism in elderly people low T3–syndrome in old age. Klin Wochenschr 1981; 59:315–23.

96. Chakraborti S, Chakraborti T, Mandal M, et al. Hypothalamic–pituitary–thyroid axis status of humans during development of ageing process. Clin Chim Acta 1999;288: 137–45.

97. Hesch RD, Husch M, Kodding R, et al. Treatment of dopamine-dependent shock with triiodothyronine. Endocr Res Commun 1981;8:299–301.

98. Klemperer JD, Klein IL, Ojamaa K, et al. Triiodothyronine therapy lowers the incidence of atrial fibrillation after cardiac operations. Ann Thorac Surg 1996;61:1323–9.

99. Smidt-Ott UM, Ascheim DD. Thyroid hormone and heart failure. Curr Heart Fail Rep 2006;3:114–9.

100. Abraham G, Milev R, Lawson JS. T3 augmentation of SSRI resistant depression. J Affect Dis 2006;91:211–5.

101. Posternak M, Novak S, Stern R, Hennessey J, Joffe R, et al. A pilot effectiveness study: placebo-controlled trial of adjunctive L-triiodothyronine (T3) used to accelerate and potentiate the antidepressant response. Int J Neuropsychopharmacol 2008;11:15–25.

102. Krotkiewski M, Holm G, Shono N. Small doses of triiodothyronine can change some risk factors associated with abdominal obesity. Int J Obes 1997;21:922–9.

103. Lowe J, Garrison R, Reichman A, Yellin J, et al. Effectiveness and safety of T3 (triiodothyronine) therapy for euthyroid fibromyalgia: a double-blind placebo-controlled response-driven crossover study. Clinical Bulletin of Myofascial Therapy 1997;2:31–58.

104. Yellin BA, Reichman AJ, Lowe JC, et al. The process of change during T3 treatment for euthyroid fibromyalgia: a double-blind placebo-controlled crossover study. In: The Metabolic Treatment of Fibromyalgia. Old Fort (NC): McDowell Publishing; 2000.

105. Tanis BC, Westendorp RGJ, Smelt AHM. Effect of thyroid substitution on hypercholesterolaemia in patients with subclinical hypothyroidism: a re-analysis of intervention studies. Clin Endocrinol 1996;44:643–9.

Diets for Successful Aging

Carol C. Ziegler, MS, RD, MSN*, Mohamad A. Sidani, MD, MS

KEYWORDS

- Aging • Longevity • Diet • Nutrition • Life span
- Dietary pattern • Mediterranean diet • Caloric restriction

AGING

Aging is the accumulation of biological changes over time leading to decreased biological functioning and impaired ability to adapt to stressors.[1] Evolving theories on the aging process have been reviewed extensively in the literature and it is well established that the rate of aging is determined by a combination of genetic and environmental factors.[2,3] It is theorized that chronic disease contributes to the aging process by speeding the rate and accumulation of damaging biological changes.[4] Many interventions that slow the progression of age-related illness also slow the rate of aging.[5] The significant age-related illnesses are cardiovascular disease (CVD), cerebrovascular disease, cancer, age-associated cognitive decline, and musculoskeletal degeneration owing to sarcopenia and osteoporosis.[6] These chronic conditions significantly contribute to age-related morbidity and dietary pattern plays a significant role in their progression.

Successful aging is defined by the compression of morbidity toward the attainment of maximal life expectancy free of age-related disease.[7] Maximum life expectancy for humans is about 122 years,[8–10] and the average life expectancy is around 85 years.[7,9,10] Since the mid 1800s, human life expectancy has increased by approximately 2.5 years per decade and this increase is accompanied by an increase in health span, or disease-free years.[11] In developed nations, increasing trends in health expectancy follow similar increases in total life expectancy.[12–14] Humans seem to be enjoying compressed morbidity—increasing life span with longer periods in a disease-free state. However, great health disparity and variations exist across populations regarding longevity and life expectancy.[15] This article discusses dietary patterns that have been linked with maximal life expectancy (longevity), successful aging, and the prevention of the aforementioned age-related diseases. Effects of specific nutrients on aging processes are discussed in other articles.

Meharry Medical College, Department of Family and Community Medicine, 1005 Dr. D. B. Todd Jr. Blvd., Nashville, TN 37208, USA
* Corresponding author.
E-mail address: cziegler@mmc.edu

Clin Geriatr Med 27 (2011) 577–589
doi:10.1016/j.cger.2011.07.005
0749-0690/11/$ – see front matter © 2011 Elsevier Inc. All rights reserved.

geriatric.theclinics.com

with the metabolic syndrome.[68–75] A recent meta-analysis revealed that 35 randomized controlled trials, 2 prospective studies, and 13 cross-sectional studies showed an association between adherence to the Mediterranean diet and decreases in blood glucose, blood pressure, and triglyceride levels.[76]

Mediterranean diet and ARCD

ARCD contributes significantly to disability and diminished longevity in the aging population. Essential fatty acids have been demonstrated to be critical in cognitive function in animal studies.[77,78] Significant links between diet and ARCD have been demonstrated in humans as well. In a multiethnic community-based study, a dose-dependent relationship was found between adherence to the Mediterranean diet and decreases in ARCD, Alzheimer's disease, and mortality from Alzheimer's disease.[79,80] The recent Italian Longitudinal Study on Aging concluded that diets high in MUFA and PUFA, like the Mediterranean diet, are associated with improved cognition in the elderly.[81–84] The researchers attributed these effects to improved structural integrity of neuronal cell membranes with higher intakes of MUFA. This accumulating evidence suggests a possible role for the Mediterranean diet pattern in prevention of ARCD.

Mediterranean diet and cancer

Cancer rates increase sharply with advancing age.[85] Malignancy is the second leading cause of death in elderly persons, after heart disease.[86] Diet is a significant and preventable cause of cancer-related death in the United States.[87] It also may be linked to the initiation and progression of up to 38% of preventable cancer incidence.[87] Longitudinal studies have demonstrated a link between strict adherence to the Mediterranean diet and decrease in the risk of death from cancer.[76] The European Prospective Investigation into Cancer and Nutrition, a cohort study, linked moderate alcohol intake and increased consumption of fruits, nuts, and legumes with decreased cancer-related mortality.[54,60,74] A 4-year follow-up of the Lyon diet heart study showed a protective effect of the dietary pattern against cancers.[72]

Few studies have addressed the effects of the Mediterranean diet on cancer prevention. A case-control study showed no beneficial effect of this dietary pattern on breast cancer prevention.[88] More research is needed to determine the effects of adherence to the Mediterranean diet on specific types of cancer and their prevention, initiation, promotion, and progression. The Mediterranean diet provides a framework for creating desirable macronutrient profiles and there is good evidence that adhering to this type of diet may promote increases in health span through prevention of cardiometabolic diseases associated with aging.

Diets of Centenarians: Okinawa

The people of Okinawa, Japan, are known worldwide for their longevity and impressive health span. Boasting the greatest number of centenarians in the world, the average life expectancy at birth on the island is around 81.2 years and many researchers believe that the diet of Okinawa, in addition to the genetic makeup and lifestyle of the islanders, may contribute to their longevity.[89,90] Adults living in Okinawa have significantly decreased risk for cancer (69%), stroke (59%), and heart disease (59%) relative to the rest of the population of Japan.[91] At the time of the initial study by Kagawa,[89] total energy intake for adults on the island was about 20% less than the average Japanese caloric intake. Protein and fat intakes were roughly equivalent between islanders and the mainland Japanese population during the same period, suggesting that sources of dietary fat and carbohydrate likely played a significant role in dietary differences between the 2 groups. (Protein sources remained relatively constant between geographic regions).

Investigations into the dietary patterns of Okinawa revealed that the traditional diet of Okinawa is nutritionally similar to the Mediterranean and Dietary Approaches to Stop Hypertension diets. The Okinawa dietary pattern is characterized by large quantities of spices and herbs that may be termed "functional foods."[90] The diet incorporates high intakes of fiber and antioxidants, and lower intakes of saturated fat, high glycemic foods, and calories.[90] This dietary composition may be contributing to the low rates of CVD and longevity enjoyed by the Okinawans. In 1978, Kagawa predicted that changes in the traditional Okinawan culture and the westernization of dietary practices would likely decrease the number of centenarians in that population.[89] As Okinawans move from the island to the mainland, their mortality rates approach those of their mainland counterparts.[91] Although Okinawa provides a unique picture of the potential role of diet in longevity, more research is needed to determine the individual contributions of lifestyle, and environmental and genetic factors to the health span and longevity of this population.

Vegetarian Diets

The repeating motif of plant-based diets and population longevity has led to investigations into the effects of increased fruit and vegetable consumption on mortality. There is good evidence to suggest that a plant-based diet, high in fruits and vegetables, is protective against age-related illnesses. In Japan, a longitudinal study of elderly people demonstrated that increased intake of fruits, vegetables, seaweed, and soy products was inversely correlated with all-cause mortality.[92] Similar results were observed in a cohort study demonstrating that a traditional Japanese diet rich in fruits, vegetables, fish, and soy products decreased CVD mortality in adults.[93] Increased intake of fruits and vegetables was associated with decreases in CVD mortality in several observational cohort studies.[94,95] In 2002, the World Health Organization reported that a diet poor in fruits and vegetables is the third preventable risk factor for chronic diseases including, CVD, cerebrovascular diseases and cancers.[96]

A common thread among dietary patterns, longevity, and decreased incidence of age-related chronic diseases is the relatively high proportional intake of plant-based foods. In the following discussion on vegetarian diets and age-related diseases the term vegetarian is loosely defined and represents various plant-based eating patterns. Also, many vegetarians have adopted numerous health-promoting behaviors that may also contribute to observed health effects.[97]

Vegetarian diets seem to offer protection against obesity, hypertension, CVD, and type 2 diabetes.[97,98] Loma Linda, California, the home of a large percentage of Seventh Day Adventists boasts one of the highest ratios of centenarians in the world.[98] One longitudinal study investigating the effects of vegetarian diets on longevity followed a cohort of Seventh Day Adventists for 21 years.[98,99] The authors report that persons with predominantly vegetarian eating patterns had lower age-associated mortality rates, lower rates of coronary heart disease, but equivalent rates of cancer relative to nonvegetarian Seventh Day Adventists. A national cohort study reported significant reduction in all-cause mortality in persons following a vegetarian diet.[100]

High-Protein, Low-Carbohydrate Diets

Sarcopenia is a significant cause of disability in the elderly.[101] Adopting a more sedentary lifestyle is linked to the development of sarcopenia.[101] However, the role of dietary protein in the prevention of age-related musculoskeletal decline is not clearly defined. Short-term studies suggest that increasing dietary protein may be beneficial in maintaining muscle mass in the elderly.[102,103] However, at present there are no long-term studies quantifying the benefits of protein supplementation versus the risks of impaired renal function and no recommendations regarding specific levels of protein supplementation to prevent sarcopenia in the elderly. Although there is no evidence to suggest that a moderate increase in protein intake would increase the risk for renal impairment in healthy persons, renal function may decrease with aging and high protein intakes are contraindicated in persons with renal dysfunction. At present, it is prudent to recommend resistance exercise training and adequate protein intake in the elderly. More research is needed to determine specific sources and levels of protein supplementation to prevent sarcopenia in the elderly.

The high-protein diet has been suggested as an antidote to aging and obesity-related diseases. Meals with high glycemic load result in activation of the insulin-signaling pathways with downstream increases in proinflammatory mediators a condition associated with CVDs.[104,105] High-protein/low-carbohydrate diets such as the Atkins diet, demonstrate short-term health benefits of weight loss. However, there are no long-term clinical studies to substantiate the claim that these diets may decrease CVDs.[106,107] No human studies were found demonstrating effects of high-protein diets on lifespan.

Caloric Restriction

Caloric restriction involves reduction of caloric intake (approximately 30%–40% from baseline) while maintaining high dietary quality, free of nutrient deficiencies.[108] Caloric restriction as a means of slowing aging first became a topic of interest during the depression in the 1930s.[109] Contrary to scientific prediction that hunger would reduce lifespan, lifespan seemed to increase during the great depression, leading scientists to question the role of caloric intake in human longevity.

Caloric restriction in experimental models has traditionally been defined as a 40% decrease in caloric intake compared with subjects fed ad libitum. In the 1930s, McCay et al[110] demonstrated that caloric restriction could slow the aging process, postpone age-related illness and extend lifespan of laboratory rats by up to 100%. Since then, caloric restriction has been demonstrated to effectively slow aging and extend lifespan in numerous animal species such as the fruit flies, earthworms, yeast, mice, rats, and dogs.[1] Research in primate models has demonstrated that restricting caloric intake while maintaining nutrient density lengthens the lifespan of adults compared with their ad libitum–fed counterparts.[109]

Spontaneous data collection on effects of caloric restriction in humans resulted from a planning error during the Biosphere 2 experiment and 8 participants in the experiment had to drastically reduce their caloric intakes for 2 years. Physiologic changes observed in the participants included weight loss and decreases in insulin, blood pressure, and cholesterol levels.[111] These effects are also seen in rodent and primate models of caloric restriction,[112] but are not predictive of increased longevity in humans. Short-term caloric restriction for 6 months decreased fasting insulin level and core body temperature in humans in a randomized, controlled trial.[113] Caloric restriction of 6 years reduced risk for atherosclerosis and improved diastolic heart function in humans as demonstrated in several randomized controlled trials.[114–116]

These results combine to present a promising picture of the potential of caloric restriction in human lifespan extension. However, when caloric restriction occurs naturally in humans it is often in the context of poor dietary quality and additional external pressures and, therefore, is accompanied by poor health outcomes.[117]

Molecular research shows that under harsh environmental conditions, such as scarcity of food, physiologic processes shift from growth and reproduction toward protection and maintenance.[5] Experts theorize that this shift may promote extended lifespan.[5] At present, these conclusions are theoretically based and research into the effects of caloric restriction is only just beginning.

Caloric restriction in the elderly: special concerns

Although caloric restriction is promising, evidence from the National Health and Nutrition Examination Survey-II Epidemiological Follow-up study shows that decreased food intake and weight loss in elderly is associated with poor health outcomes and increased mortality.[118] The notion that caloric restriction extends human life span is inconclusive at this time.

THE OPTIMAL DIET FOR SUCCESSFUL AGING

Although we have clear evidence for the role of diet in age-related diseases, definitive evidence delineating the ultimate diet for slowing the aging process and maximizing longevity is lacking. Epidemiologic studies link longevity with dietary patterns that are high in fruits and vegetables, and lower in saturated fats, meats, dairy products, refined grains, and sweets; the Mediterranean-type diet provides a framework for achieving these parameters.

Results emerging from caloric restriction studies in animal models are promising, but it is premature to recommend caloric restriction at this time. Caloric restriction is contraindicated in the elderly. Recommending that patients maintain an active lifestyle, avoid obesity, reduce intake of sweets and simple carbohydrates, maximize intake of fruits and vegetables, and aim for a higher proportion of dietary fat from PUFA, MUFA and omega 3 fatty acids, while limiting saturated fats, is good practice at this time.

Establishing good experimental controls in aging research is difficult, because researchers are still determining reliable biomarkers of the aging process. In looking at epidemiologic evidence, causal relationships cannot be drawn and factors such as toxin exposure, stress, community, and exercise likely play a significant role in the aging process. It is unlikely that in the current health environment, dietary interventions will increase life expectancy to the same degree that medical technological advances have altered it since the 1960s.

REFERENCES

1. Massoro EJ. Concepts and hypothesis of basic aging process. In: Byung Pal Yu, editor. Free Radicals in Aging. Boca Raton (FL): CRC Press; 1993. p. 1–9.
2. Ljubuncic P, Reznick A. The evolutionary theories of aging revisited: a mini-review. Gerontology 2009;55:205–16.
3. Harman D. Aging: phenomena and theories. Ann NY Acad Sci 1998;854:1–7.
4. Blumenthal HT. The aging-disease dichotomy: true or false? J Gerontol A Biol Sci Med Sci 2003;58:138–45.
5. Kenyon C. The genetics of aging. Nature 2010;464:504–12.
6. Lopez A, Mathers C, Ezzati M, et al. Global and regional burden of disease and risk factors, 2001: systematic analysis of population health data. Lancet 2006;367: 1747–57.
7. Fries JF. 1988. Aging, natural death and the compression of morbidity. N Engl J Med 1998;303:130–5.
8. Harman D. Aging: prospects for further increases in the functional lifespan. Age 1994;17:119–46.

9. Woodhall B, Joblon S. Prospects for future increases in average longevity. Geriatrics 1957;12:586–91.

10. Olshansky S, Carnes B, Cassel C. In search of Methuselah: estimating the upper limits to human longevity. Science 1990;250:634–40.

11. Christensen K, McGue M, Petersen I, et al. Exceptional longevity does not result in excessive levels of disability. Proc Natl Acad Sci U S A 2008;105:13274–9.

12. Jeune B, Bronnum-Hansen H. Trends in health expectancy at age 65 for various health indicators, 1987–2005, Denmark. Eur J Aging 2008;5:279–85.

13. Cambois E, Clavel A, Romieu I, et al. Trends in disability-free life expectancy at age 65 in France: consistent and diverging patterns according to the underlying disability measure. Eur J Aging 2008;5:287–98.

14. Kristjuhan U. Youth maintenance and postponing human aging in reality. Rejuvenation Res 2008;11:505–8.

15. Murray CJ, Kulkarni SC, Michaud C, et al. Eight Americas: Investigating mortality disparities across races, counties and race-counties in the United States. PLoS Med 2006;3:e260.

16. Hu FB. Dietary pattern analysis: a new direction in nutritional epidemiology. Curr Opin Lipidol 2002;13:3–9.

17. Zarraga IG, Schwarz ER. Impact of dietary patterns and interventions on cardiovascular health. Circulation 2006;114:961–73.

18. Fung TT, Willett WC, Stampfer MJ, et al. Dietary patterns and the risk of coronary heart disease in women. Arch Intern Med 2001;161:1857–62.

19. Fung TT, Stampfer MJ, Manson JE, et al. Prospective study of major dietary patterns and stroke risk in women. Stroke 2004;35:2014–9.

20. Schulze M, Fung TT, Manson JE, et al. Dietary patterns and changes in body weight in women. Obesity (Silver Spring) 2006;14:1444–53.

21. Fung TT, Schulze M, Manson JE, et al. Dietary patterns, meat intake, and the risk of type 2 diabetes in women. Arch Intern Med 2004;164:2235–40.

22. Fung T, Hu FB, Fuchs C, et al. Major dietary patterns and risk of colorectal cancer in women. Arch Intern Med 2003;163:309–14.

23. Heidemann C, Schulze M, Franco O, et al. Dietary pattern: risk and mortality from cardiovascular disease, cancer, and all causes in a prospective cohort of women. Circulation 2008;118;230–7.

24. Colditz GA, Hankinson SE. The Nurses' Health Study: lifestyle and health among women. Nat Rev Cancer 2005;5:388–96.

25. Lopez-Garcia E, Schulze MB, Fung TT, et al. Major dietary patterns are related to plasma concentrations of markers of inflammation and endothelial dysfunction. Am J Clin Nutr 2004;80:1029–35.

26. Eaton SB, Konner MJ. Paleolithic nutrition. A consideration of its nature and current implications. N Engl J Med 1985;312:283–9.

27. Eaton SB, Konner M, Shostack M. Stone agers in the fast lane: chronic degenerative diseases in evolutionary perspective. Am J Med 1988;84:739–49.

28. Cordain L, Watkins B, Florant G, et al. Fatty acid analysis of wild ruminant tissues: evolutionary implications for reducing diet-related chronic disease. Eur J Clin Nutr 2002;56:181–91.

29. Cordain L, Eaton S, Sebastian A, et al. Origins and evolution of the western diet: health implications for the twenty-first century. Am J Clin Nutr 2005;81:341–54.

30. Yudkin J. Sugar and disease. Nature 1972;239:197–9.

31. Yudkin J, Szanto S. The relationship between sucrose intake, plasma insulin and platelet adhesiveness in men with and without occlusive arteriosclerosis. Proc Nutr Soc 1970;28(Suppl):2A–3A.

32. Liu S, Willett WC. Dietary glycemic load and atherothrombotic risk. Curr Atheroscler Rep 2002;4:454–61.
33. Ludwig D. The glycemic index: physiological mechanisms relating obesity, diabetes, and cardiovascular disease. JAMA 2002;287:2414–23.
34. Cordain L, Eades MR, Eades MD. Hyperinsulinemic diseases of civilization: more than just syndrome X. Comp Biochem Physiol A Mol Integr Physiol 2003;136:95–112.
35. Reaven GM. Pathophysiology of insulin resistance in human disease. Physiol Rev 1995;75:473–86.
36. DeLorgeril M, Salen P, Martin J, et al. Mediterranean diet, traditional risk factors, and the rate of cardiovascular complications after myocardial infarction: final report of the Lyon Diet Heart Study. Circulation 1999;99:779–85.
37. Von Schacky C, Angerer P, Kothny W, et al. The effect of omega-3 fatty acids on coronary atherosclerosis. A randomized, double-blind, placebo-controlled trial. Ann Intern Med 1999;130:554–62.
38. Kris-Etherton PM, Taylor DS, Yu-Poth S, et al. Polyunsaturated fatty acids in the food chain in the United States. Am J Clin Nutr 2000;71:179S–88S.
39. Kris-Etherton PM, Hecker KD, Binkoski AE. Polyunsaturated fatty acids and cardiovascular health. Nutr Rev 2004;62:414–26.
40. Rule DC, Broughton KS, Shellito SM, et al. Comparison of muscle fatty acid profiles and cholesterol concentrations of bison, beef, cattle, elk and chicken. J Anim Sci 2002;80:1202–11.
41. Osler M, Heitmann BL, Gerdes LU, et al. Dietary patterns and mortality in Danish men and women: a prospective observational study. Br J Nutr 2001;85:219–25.
42. Kroenke CH, Fung TT, Hu FB, et al. Dietary patterns and survival after breast cancer diagnosis. J Clin Oncol 2005;23:9295–303.
43. Pierce JP, Natarajan L, Caan BJ, et al. Influence of a diet very high in vegetables, fruit, and fiber and low in fat on prognosis following treatment for breast cancer: the Women's Healthy Eating and Living (WHEL) randomized trial. JAMA 2007; 298:289–98.
44. Kannel WB, Kannel C, Paffenbarger RS Jr, et al. Heart rate and cardiovascular mortality: the Framingham Study. Am Heart J 1987;113:1489–94.
45. Appel LJ, Moore TJ, Obarzenek E, et al. A clinical trial of the effects of dietary pattern on blood pressure. N Engl J Med 1997;336:1117–24.
46. Gross L, Li L, Ford ES, et al. Increased consumption of refined carbohydrates and the epidemic of type 2 diabetes in the United States: an ecologic assessment. Am J Clin Nutr 2004;79:774–9.
47. Keys A, Menotti A, Karoven MJ. The diet and the 15-year death rate in the seven countries study. Am J Epidemiol 1986;124:903–15.
48. Petroni A, Blasevich M, Salami M, et al. Inhibition of platelet aggregation and eicosanoid production by phenolic compounds of olive oil. Thrombos Res 1995;78: 151–60.
49. Masala G, Ceroti M, Pala V, et al. A dietary pattern rich in olive oil and raw vegetables is associated with lower mortality in Italian elderly subjects. Br J Nutr 2007;98:406–15.
50. Mattson FH, Grundy SM. Comparison of effects of dietary saturated, monounsaturated and polyunsaturated fatty acids on plasma lipids and lipoproteins. J Lipid Res 1985;26:194–202.
51. Visioli F, Bellomo G, Montedoro G, et al. Low density lipoprotein oxidation is inhibited in vitro by olive oil constituents. Atherosclerosis 1995;117:25–32.

93. Shimazu T, Kuriyama S, Hozawa A, et al. Dietary patterns and cardiovascular disease mortality in Japan: a prospective cohort study. Int J Epidemiol 2007;36: 600–9.

94. He FJ, Nowson CA, MacGregor GA. Fruit and vegetable consumption and stroke: meta-analysis of cohort studies. Lancet 2006;367:320–6.

95. Dauchet L, Amouyel P, Hercberg S, et al. Fruit and vegetable consumption and risk of coronary heart disease: a meta-analysis of cohort studies. J Nutr 2006; 136:2588–93.

96. World health report 2002. Reducing Risks, Promoting Healthy Life. World Health Organization. Available at: http://www.who.int/whr/2002/en/whr02_en.pdf. Accessed March 28, 2011.

97. Dwyer JT. Health aspects of vegetarian diets. Am J Clin Nutr 1988;48:712–38.

98. Kahn HA, Phillips RL, Snowdon DA, et al. Association between reported diet and all cause mortality: twenty-one year follow-up on 27,530 adult Seventh Day Adventists. Am J Epidemiol 1984;119:775–87.

99. Fraser G. Diet, life expectancy and chronic disease: studies of Seventh Day Adventists and other vegetarians. New York: Oxford University Press; 1988.

100. Kant AK, Graubard BI, Schatzkin A. Dietary patterns predict mortality in a national cohort: the National Health Interview Surveys, 1987 and 1992. J Nutr 2004;134: 1793–9.

101. Volpi E, Nazami R, Fujita S. Muscle tissue changes with aging. Curr Opin Clin Nutr Metab Care 2004:7;405–10.

102. Paddon-Jones D. Interplay of stress and physical activity on muscle loss: nutritional countermeasures. J Nutr 2006:136;2123–6.

103. Paddon-Jones D, Sheffield-Moore M, Urban RJ, et al. Essential amino acid and carbohydrate supplementation ameliorates muscle protein loss in humans during 28 days bedrest. J Clin Endocrinol Metab 2004:89;4351–8.

104. Qi L, van Dam RM, Liu S, et al. Whole-grain, bran, and cereal fiber intakes and markers of systemic inflammation in diabetic women. Diabetes Care 2006;29: 207–11.

105. Kershaw EE, Flier JS. Adipose tissue as an endocrine organ. J Clin Endocrinol Metab 2004;89:2548–56.

106. Clifton PM, Keogh JB, Naokes M. Long-term effects of a high protein weight-loss diet. Am J Clin Nutr 2008;87:23–9.

107. Bravata DM, Sanders L, Huang J, et al. Efficacy and safety of low-carbohydrate diets: a systematic review. JAMA 2003;289:1837–50.

108. Tapia Granados JA, Diez Roux AV. Life and death during the great depression. Proc Natl Acad Sci U S A 2009;106:17290–5.

109. McCay CM, Crowel MF, Maynard LA. The effect of retarded growth upon the length of the life span and upon the ultimate body size. J Nutr 1935;10:63–79.

110. Lane MA, Black A, Ingram DK, et al. Calorie restriction in nonhuman primates: implications for age-related disease risk. J Anti-Aging Med 1998:1;315–26.

111. Walford RL, Mock D, Verdery R, et al. Calorie restriction in biosphere 2: alterations in physiologic, hematologic, hormonal, and biochemical parameters in humans restricted for a 2-year period. J Gerontol A Biol Sci Med Sci 2002;57:B211–24.

112. Roth GS, Lane MA, Ingram DK, et al. Biomarkers of caloric restriction may predict longevity in humans. Science 2002;297:811.

113. Heilbronn L, de Jonge L, Frisard MI, et al. Effect of 6-month calorie restriction on biomarkers of longevity, metabolic adaptation, and oxidative stress in overweight individuals: a randomized controlled trial. JAMA 2006;295:1539–48.

114. Fontana L, Meyer TE, Klein S, et al. Long term caloric restriction is highly effective in reducing the risk for atherosclerosis in humans. Proc Natl Acad Sci U S A 2004;101: 6659–63.
115. Meyer TE, Kovacs SJ, Ehsani AA, et al. Long term caloric restriction ameliorates the decline in diastolic heart function in humans. J Am Coll Cardiol 2006;47:398–402.
116. Fontana L, Klein S. Aging, adiposity and caloric restriction. JAMA 2007;297:986–94.
117. Phelan JP, Austad SN. Natural selection, dietary restriction and extended longevity. Growth Dev Aging 1989;53:4–6.
118. Sahyoun NR, Serdula MK, Galuska DA, et al. The epidemiology of recent involuntary weight loss in the United States Population. J Nutr Health Aging 2004;8:510–7.

randomized primary and secondary prevention trials, beta-carotene, vitamin A, and vitamin E all caused an increase in mortality at a rate of about 5%.[3] Although there were wide variations in the amounts of antioxidants administered in the various trials, the size of the analysis (232,606 participants) and the endpoint of all-cause mortality (which limits outcome bias) both lend credibility to these findings, and raise concern about patients using excessive doses of these vitamin supplements. In this study, vitamin C and selenium had no effect on mortality.[3]

VITAMIN A AND CAROTENOIDS

Vitamin A is a group of compounds found in animal products, the most clinically significant of which are retinol and dehydroretinol. Carotenoids are a group of hundreds of plant pigments with antioxidant activity and give fruit, vegetables, and plant materials their yellow, orange, and red coloring. Certain carotenoids, particularly beta carotene, can be efficiently made into vitamin A, and account for over half the vitamin A activity in the human body. The Recommended Daily Allowance (RDA) for vitamin A is 700 μg for females and 900 μg for males.

Vitamin A and Osteoporosis

Osteoporosis is especially common in countries where vitamin A intake is high. In a nested case-control study, vitamin A intake was associated with reduced bone mineral density and increased risk for hip fracture. Compared with intakes of 500 μg/d, no differences in bone mineral density were found with daily intakes up to 1500 μg, but bone mineral density was reduced and the risk for hip fracture doubled (odds ratio, 2.1; 95% confidence interval, 1.1–4.0) for intakes greater than 1500 μg/d. Every 1000 μg increase in daily intake of retinol increased the risk for hip fracture by 68%.[4] Women enrolled in the Nurses Health Study with daily intakes greater than 3000 μg had significantly increased risk for hip fracture compared with those consuming less than 1250 μg.[5] Beta carotenes were not associated with an increased risk of hip fractures or decreased bone density, possibly because their conversion to vitamin A decreases when body stores are full.

Beta Carotene and Cancer

In the Alpha-Tocopherol Beta-Carotene Cancer Prevention Study, a randomized controlled trial (RCT) of 29,133 male cigarette smokers, the daily intake of 20 mg of beta carotene for 5 to 8 years increased the incidence of lung cancer by 18%.[6] Another RCT, the Carotene and Retinol Efficacy Trial, showed an increase in the incidence of in cancer in subjects who took 30 mg beta carotene and 25,000 IU vitamin A daily.[7]

Beta Carotenes and Macular Degeneration

In developed countries, age-related macular degeneration (AMD) is the leading cause of blindness in older adults. In the Age-Related Eye Disease Study, a RCT in 360 patients at high risk of developing advanced stages of AMD (patients had intermediate AMD in both eyes or advanced AMD in only 1 eye), antioxidant supplements lowered the risk of progression to advanced AMD by 25% and the risk of moderate vision loss by 19%. The supplement included vitamin C 500 mg, zinc oxide 80 mg, cupric oxide 2 mg, vitamin E 400 IU, and beta carotene 15 mg.[8] Because beta carotene supplements increase the risk of developing cancer in smokers, patients taking high doses of beta carotene for AMD should be counseled about potential risks. A meta analysis study of 23,099 persons found that beta carotene (or vitamin E) supplements are not helpful in the prevention of AMD.[9]

VITAMIN C

The RDA for vitamin C is 90 mg in males and 75 mg in females. Studies on the role of vitamin C as an antioxidant in preventing cancer and cardiovascular disease have often included other antioxidants and have not shown benefit. It has had no effect on cancer or cardiovascular disease in RCTs.[10,11]

VITAMIN E

Vitamin E is a fat-soluble antioxidant. The RDA for vitamin E is 15 mg (22.4 IU) for adults. Diets high in foods rich in vitamin E are associated with a lower risk of coronary heart disease (CHD), and vitamin E reduces atherosclerotic plaque formation in mouse models.[12]

Vascular Disease

The Nurses Health Study, an observational study of approximately 90,000 women, reported in 1993 that the incidence of heart disease was 30% to 40% lower in those with the highest intakes of vitamin E, primarily from supplements,[13] and among 5133 Finnish men and women followed for a mean of 14 years, higher vitamin E intakes from food were associated with decreased mortality from CHD.[14] However, RCTs have not shown vitamin E supplements to prevent CHD. The Heart Outcomes Prevention Evaluation study demonstrated no benefit from 400 IU of vitamin E daily in almost 10,000 high-risk patients over 4.5 years,[15] nor in a follow-up (Heart Outcomes Prevention Evaluation-TOO) study of almost 4000 of the original participants who continued to take vitamin E for an additional 2.5 years. Vitamin E provided no protection against heart attacks, strokes, unstable angina, or deaths from cardiovascular disease. Participants taking vitamin E were 21% more likely to be hospitalized for heart failure.[16]

In the Physicians Health Study II, 15,000 healthy physicians greater than equal to 50 years of age were randomly assigned to receive 400 IU synthetic alpha-tocopherol every other day, 500 mg vitamin C daily, both, or placebo.[17] Over 8 years, intake of vitamin E had no effect on the incidence of major cardiovascular events, myocardial infarction (MI), stroke, or cardiovascular morality, although vitamin E use was associated with a significantly increased risk of hemorrhagic stroke. In view of findings such as these, although recommending diets high in antioxidant vitamins, the American Heart Association does not support the use of vitamin E supplements to prevent cardiovascular disease.[18]

Cognitive Decline

In 1997, a RCT of 85 patients with Alzheimer disease (AD) demonstrated significant delay in functional deterioration in those patients taking 2000 IU vitamin E daily.[19] Vitamin E consumption was also associated with less cognitive decline over 3 years in a prospective cohort study of independent elderly individuals.[20] However, there was no significant decrease in progression to AD in a RCT of 769 patients with mild cognitive impairment treated with 2000 IU/d vitamin E in 2005,[21] and authors of a 2005 meta-analysis of the dose–response relationship between vitamin E supplementation and total mortality, a study that included 135,967 participants in 19 clinical trials, concluded that high-dose vitamin E supplements (>400 IU/d) may increase all-cause mortality and should be avoided.[22]

SELENIUM

Selenium is a nonmetallic element with antioxidant properties. Plants vary in their selenium content based on the selenium content of the soil in which they are grown, and the meat from livestock contains selenium in amounts related to their selenium feed content. Unlike animals, there are no known diseases associated with selenium deficiency in humans. Selenium is needed to activate the enzyme glutathione peroxidase, which destroys the peroxides that result from the metabolism of polyunsaturated fatty acids. Unlike vitamin E, selenium supplements have not been associated with an increase in mortality.[3] Population studies suggest lower rates of disease in patients with higher consumption of selenium. In an interesting study arm of the Nurse Health Study, the selenium content of the toenail clippings of 62,641 participants did not correlate with risk of developing cancer.[23]

B VITAMINS AND FOLIC ACID

Grain products sold in the United States are fortified with thiamine (B_1), riboflavin (B_2), niacin (B_3), and, since January 1998, folic acid. Other than B_{12}, deficiencies of B vitamins are uncommon. Thiamine and pyridoxine (B_6) have been investigated but not found to be of help in preventing or treating cognitive decline.[24,25]

B Vitamins and Vascular Disease

Extrapolating from the atherosclerosis seen in young children who have extremely high levels of homocysteine as a result of inborn errors of metabolism, McCully[26] proposed that deficiencies of those B vitamins may cause homocysteine elevations that contribute to atherosclerosis. Epidemiologic data confirmed an association between elevated homocysteine levels and CHD and stroke, and authors of a large meta-analysis in 2002 suggested that a 25% lowering of homocysteine would result in a 11% decrease in CHD and a 19% decrease in stroke risk.[27] A number of well-done RCTs over the past decade have examined the effect of B vitamins on the incidence of vascular events, primarily MI and stroke.[28–33] In greater than 30,000 participants studied over 3 to 7 years, all trials were able to demonstrate successful homocysteine lowering in patients taking combinations of folic acid (0.8–2.5 mg), vitamin B_6 (25–50 mg), and vitamin B_{12} (400–1000 μg); however, all failed to show any significant benefit from B vitamin supplementation verses placebo.

Although no ill effects were reported by subjects in these trials, adverse effects were reported in 252 patients with diabetic nephropathy (minimum 300 mg/d urinary albumin excretion; median serum creatinine 1.4 mg/dL) assigned to take vitamins (B_{12} 1000 μg, B_6 25 mg, and folic acid 2.5 mg) or matching placebo for 36 months. Patients taking supplements had a faster decline in glomerular filtration rate and an increase in cardiovascular and cerebrovascular events. No clear understanding exists about the mechanism of possible adverse effect of the supplements.[34]

B Vitamins and Dementia

Observational studies have reported a direct relationship between homocysteine levels and dementia,[35] and for patients in the Framingham Study followed for 8 years, those with homocysteine levels in the highest quartile had a relative risk of developing AD more than twice that of patients in the lowest quartile.[36] However, an RCT of 276 patients given folic acid (1 mg), B6 (10 mg), and B_{12} (500 mg) for 2 years to elderly patients with elevated homocysteine levels showed no improvement in cognition over placebo.[37]

A 2007 review of RCTs showed no evidence for an effect of B vitamins on cognitive function, although trials were small and of short duration.[38] A 3-year RCT of 818 patients that same year showed subtle improvements, such as improved information processing speed and word fluency, in those treated with 0.8 mg folic acid.[39] Lowering homocysteine levels with B vitamins for 2 years did not improve cognition in older men over 8 years of follow-up.[40]

B Vitamins and Cancer

Although consumption of foods high in folic acid is linked with a decrease in risk of cancer of the colon, pancreas, esophagus, and stomach, folic acid may also promote tumor growth, and recognition that folic acid increases growth of existing tumors has led to the development of folate antagonists for cancer treatment. This dual effect has been demonstrated in a mouse model of colorectal cancer (CRC), where folic acid suppresses cancer incidence, but once a neoplasm has developed, enhances cancer progression.[41]

Similarly, although epidemiologic evidence shows that a high intake of folate is associated with a lower risk of colorectal polyps and cancer, RCTs have not shown folic acid supplements to protect against colorectal adenomas.[42,43] In 1 of these studies, as in the mouse model of cancer, larger and more histologically advanced lesions were observed in patients taking folic acid.[43,44] Similarly, serum levels of B vitamins are inversely associated with the risk of lung cancer,[44] but an increase (hazard ratio, 1.21; confidence interval, 1.03–1.41) in lung cancer was seen in 2 RCTs in patients taking folate and B_{12} supplements.[45]

Vitamin B_{12}

Vitamin B_{12} is found in foods of animal origin, such as meat, eggs, and dairy products, and in vitamin-fortified foods. The RDA for B_{12} is 2.4 μg for adults, and the median dietary intake in the United States is between 4 and 6 μg. Multivitamin supplements contain between 6 and 50 μg. Deficiency of B_{12} is common. Estimates place its overall prevalence in the United States at 10% to 15% of older adults. Although most patients with low levels are asymptomatic, B_{12} deficiency can cause a wide array of cognitive, psychiatric, and neurologic symptoms and signs, any of which may be seen in the absence of anemia or macrocytosis.[46] Because high levels of folic acid can mask the hematologic manifestations of B_{12} deficiency, it may be that fewer patients are presenting with hematologic abnormalities than before grain supplementation with folic acid.[47]

Deficiency

The vitamin B_{12} absorption process is complex, and so deficiency is usually caused by perturbations of this process. Most deficiency in older adults is due to food-cobalamin malabsorption, a term that describes the malabsorption that occurs because of failure of B_{12} from food sources to be released from the proteins to which it is bound.[48] Primarily this occurs from loss of parietal cell activity that accompanies aging, but may be owing to prior partial gastrectomy, treatment with H2 blockers and proton pump inhibitors, and atrophic gastritis from alcohol abuse and *Helicobacter pylori* infection. Because B_{12} contained in vitamin supplements is not protein bound, it can effectively treat food-cobalamin malabsorption. Pernicious anemia is an uncommon cause of B_{12} deficiency in elderly patients, accounting for only 1% to 3% of cases.

Patients taking metformin may also be at risk for B_{12} deficiency. Although symptomatic deficiency was not observed, the prevalence of low B_{12} levels (<300 pg/mL) rose from 9.5% to 28.1% over 4 years an RCT of patients taking metformin 850 mg 3 times daily.[49]

Treatment and prevention

Normally, about 70% of dietary B_{12} is absorbed, but even in the absence of intrinsic factor about 1% is passively absorbed, and numerous studies have now documented the effectiveness of oral treatment, usually in daily doses of 500 to 1000 μg, even in patients with pernicious anemia.[50] No studies demonstrate the merit of giving B_{12} supplements to prevent B_{12} deficiency. However, unlike the case for many vitamins, high doses of B_{12} have not been reported to cause harm, and doses as high as 30 mg/d, 10,000 times the RDA, have been reported to be safe.[51]

VITAMIN D

Because vitamin D is manufactured in the skin and circulates through the bloodstream to stimulate receptors in other organs, it is in fact a hormone. Its synthesis depends on exposure to ultraviolet light; therefore, the high prevalence of this hormone deficiency, along with an increasing human dependence on oral sources of vitamin D, is not unexpected.[52]

Current Intake

The average adult in the United States currently consumes 260 to 360 IU, yet vitamin-replete middle-aged men in Nebraska utilize approximately 4,000 IU/d.[53] For those with little sun exposure, such as elderly patients living indoors, there exists a potential for deficiency. Currently the Institute of Medicine recommends adults ages 51 to 70 ingest 600 IU vitamin D daily, and for those over age 70, the recommendation is 800 IU. The Canadian Task Force recommends 400 to 800 IU for postmenopausal women. In addition to obtaining vitamin D through dietary sources, Health Canada recommends that all adults greater than 50 consume a 400 IU supplement each day.[54]

Physiology

Vitamin D is a group of related sterol hormones, 2 of which are clinically relevant: Ergocalciferol (D_2), produced in plants, and cholecalciferol (D_3), formed in human skin. Vitamin D, whether ingested or manufactured, is transported to the liver where it undergoes 25-α-hydroxylation. The resultant 25-hydroxy-cholecalciferol [25(OH)D], also known as calcidiol, is the most prevalent form of the vitamin in serum, and serum levels correlate with vitamin status. Circulating 25(OH) D undergoes 1-α-hydroxylation to 1,25(OH)$_2$D (calcitriol) in the kidney, which regulates bone and calcium homeostasis. Indeed, 1-α-hydroxylation occurs in other tissues, and when it does, activated 1,25(OH)$_2$D enters the nuclei of those cells, binding to vitamin D receptors and activating gene transcription and protein synthesis. This autocrine system, in which 1,25(OH)$_2$D binds to receptors in the same cells in which it is formed, is present in many tissues, and explains how a low circulating 25(OH)D substrate may have negative health consequences outside the skeletal system.[55]

Normal Serum Levels

Vitamin D status correlates with serum levels of 25(OH)D, and is defined by the inverse relationship that exists between 25(OH)D levels and parathyroid hormone (PTH). Patients with frank vitamin D deficiency have elevated PTH levels that fall with vitamin D replacement. At a 25(OH)D level of 20 ng/mL, PTH levels normalize, although they continue to decline within the normal range up to a level about 30 ng/mL. Based on this evidence, 25(OH)D levels of less than 20 ng/mL are classified as "deficient," levels of 21 to 30 ng/mL as "insufficient," and levels greater than 30 ng/mL "sufficient." Although there is consensus that levels greater than 30 ng/mL are desirable for optimal bone health and calcium homeostasis, patients who most clearly benefit from supplementation are those with levels less than 20 ng/mL. There is some evidence that serum levels as high as 36 to 40 ng/mL may be desirable for optimal function in other areas, such as fall and cancer prevention.[56]

Deficiency

Using these criteria, low levels of vitamin D are common in the United States, affecting up to one third of healthy adults and one half of medical inpatients. Groups at particular risk are persons living in the northern half of the United States (because of less sunlight exposure), and persons of color, because melanin competes with ultraviolet B photons so less vitamin D is produced in the skin. Obese individuals are at increased risk, probably because fat-soluble vitamin D is sequestered in adipose tissue and less is available for circulation.[57]

Fracture Prevention

Conflicting data on the effectiveness of vitamin D in reducing the incidence of fractures in elderly patients has been addressed by a 2005 meta-analysis of RCTs, which concluded that the ability of vitamin D to prevent nonvertebral fractures is dose dependent, and that the failure of prior trials to show improvement in fracture rates was because of a failure to analyze fracture rates in relation to vitamin D dose. The analysis, which included 5 RCTs for hip fracture (9294 patients) and 7 RCTs for nonvertebral fracture (9820 patients), demonstrated that, compared with placebo, there was a 26% decrease in hip fractures, and a 23% decrease in nonvertebral fractures in patients prescribed 700 to 800 IU of vitamin D daily. Patients prescribed 400 IU daily had no reduction in fracture risk.[58] Follow-up meta-analysis by the same authors involving greater than 40,000 patients 4 years later showed similar findings. Whether or not patients were prescribed calcium supplements did not seem to affect fracture rates.[59]

Falls

The magnitude of the effect of vitamin D on falls is similar to its effect on fracture risk, with a decrease of about 20% in those taking 800 IU vitamin D daily.[60] A meta-analysis of 8 RCTs involving 2426 patients demonstrated a 23% decrease in fall risk for patients who achieved a serum 25(OH)D level of greater than equal to 24 ng/mL.[61] Currently, less than 9% of older adults have serum levels greater than 36 ng/mL, yet measurements of lower extremity function continue to increase up to levels this high.[62] There are no RCTs showing that supplementing patients to achieve vitamin D levels this high is more effective at preventing falls than simply adding an 800 IU vitamin D supplement.

Cancer Prevention

Epidemiologic evidence suggests an inverse relationship between the incidence of CRC and both intake and serum levels of vitamin D, and authors of a 2007 meta-analysis suggested that increasing daily intake of vitamin D to 1000 to 2000 IU daily could reduce the risk of CRC.[63] Others suggest optimal CRC prevention from levels of 25(OH)D of greater than equal to 36 ng/mL.[64] However, RCTs have not yet demonstrated the effectiveness of vitamin D in CRC prevention.[65,66]

Cardiovascular Disease

No decrease in cardiovascular morbidity or mortality was observed in patients taking 400 IU vitamin D_3 in the Women's Health Initiative, although this dose of vitamin D was lower than that required to demonstrate other positive health outcomes.[67] Other observational studies suggest a protective role for higher serum levels of vitamin D in cardiovascular disease. In 13,331 people participating in the Third National Health and Nutrition Examination Survey followed for 6 to 12 years, 25(OH)D levels correlated inversely with mortality.[68] A nested case-control study of 18,225 men enrolled in the Health Professionals Follow-Up Study demonstrated that, over 10 years, the risk for MI and fatal MI in men with 25(OH)D levels less than 15 ng/mL was twice that of men with levels greater than 30 ng/mL,[69] and participants in the Framingham Offspring Study with low 25(OH)D levels had a 53% to 80% higher incidence of combined cardiovascular endpoints (MI, stroke, congestive heart failure) over 5 years.[70] However, there are no RCTs demonstrating positive cardiovascular outcomes from vitamin D supplementation, and some data suggest that vitamin D could advance atherogenesis in certain populations.[71]

Other Health Outcomes

Vitamin D lowers blood pressure slightly,[72] and may improve musculoskeletal pain.[73] A meta-analysis of 57,000 patients taking 300 to 2000 IU vitamin D daily suggest total mortality may be decreased by supplements.[74]

Safety

Although vitamin D intoxication from oral intake is known to occur, it is uncommon. The Institute of Medicine lists the tolerable upper limit as 2000 IU/d, but daily doses of 10,000 IU have been given to patients for 5 months without any sign of intoxication.[75] To assess both the effectiveness and safety of patients being given vitamin D supplements, serum 25(OH)D levels can be monitored. Most reports of hypercalcemia have occurred at levels greater than 300 ng/mL, and toxicity has not been seen with levels less than 150 ng/mL.[76] Caution should be exercised in patients with sarcoidosis and other chronic granulomatous diseases, who may develop hypercalcemia when 25(OH)D levels rise above 30 ng/mL. These patients have significant increase and activation of macrophages, which have 1-α-hydroxylase activity that is insensitive to PTH feedback.

Supplementation

Because vitamin D is not commonly found in many foods, to meet Institute of Medicine goals most patients need oral supplements. Although a serving (3.5 oz) of fresh, wild-caught salmon contains 600 to 1000 IU of vitamin D_3, and servings of canned tuna, salmon, or sardines each contain between 250 and 600 IU, vitamin D is found naturally in large amounts (>100 IU per serving) in very few other foods. Because of fortification, in the United States there are about 100 IU of vitamin D in an 8-oz serving of milk. Vitamin D-fortified orange juice, yogurt, cheese, and breakfast cereal can each contain up to 100 IU per serving. Vitamin D_3 can be purchased without prescription in doses up to 2000 IU. Prescription vitamin D comes as vitamin D_2 in a dose of 50,000 IU. There may be a more robust response in serum levels when treating patients with D_3 compared with comparable doses of D_2.[77]

   Patients with frank deficiency are treated with 50,000 IU vitamin D_2 weekly for 8 to 12 weeks. Patients without frank deficiency can take vitamin supplements in doses of 400 to 2000 IU/d. In general, serum 25(OH)D levels will rise about 1 ng/mL for every

100 IU of oral supplement, and serum levels can be monitored a few months after initiating supplementation. Alternatively, institutionalized patients can empirically be given 800 IU/d, because this is the dose that has been most studied and shown in RCTs to lower both fracture and fall rates.

For compliance reasons, patients may be prescribed 50,000 IU semi-monthly to every other month. A dose of 100,000 IU every 4 months was effective in lowering both hip fracture and mortality over 5 years.[78] However, an RCT involving 2256 elderly women at high risk for hip fracture who were treated with 500,000 IU once yearly for 3 to 5 years showed a 15% increase in falls, and a 26% increase in fractures compared with placebo. Falls tended to occur within the 3 months after the annual vitamin D administration. The reasons for this unexpected increase in falls are unknown.[79]

CALCIUM

An adequate calcium intake throughout life may lessen the risk of osteoporosis, and the US Food and Drug Administration has authorized that calcium supplement labeling (along with vitamin D) may include a health claim regarding osteoporosis prevention. The current RDA for calcium is 1200 mg of elemental calcium daily for adults greater than 50 years of age. About 25% of adults in the United States ingest this much calcium.[5]

Through efficient handling of calcium, adults are able to maintain calcium balance over a wide range of calcium intakes. A 2007 review of carefully conducted studies on calcium balance by the US Department of Agriculture estimated that a daily intake of 741 mg would maintain calcium balance for healthy adults, and suggested the RDA for calcium of only 1035 mg/d, lower than the current 1200 mg.[80] Although calcium carbonate is the most commonly consumed calcium supplement, calcium citrate is more reliably absorbed in achlorhydric patients, and so may be more effectively absorbed in the elderly. Calcium carbonate contains 40% elemental calcium and calcium citrate 21%.

In addition to lessening the likelihood for osteoporosis and fracture, higher calcium intakes are variably associated with lower risks for hypertension and colon cancer.[81] An RCT of 930 patients given supplements of 1200 mg elemental calcium showed a modest 20% decrease in recurrent adenomas that extended for years after the trail ended.[82] Although patients in the Women's Health Initiative had a higher risk of kidney stones on 1000 mg of calcium and 400 IU vitamin D daily, other studies (RCTs or cohort) show a decrease in risk.[83]

There is an association between high intakes of dairy products and dietary calcium and prostate cancer[84]; however this association is likely due to the effect of dairy proteins on insulin-like growth-factor I, and not calcium itself.[85]

Studies examining the relationship between calcium intake and cardiovascular disease have generally shown no association. In Japan, because of a lower intake of dairy products, calcium intakes are significantly lower than in the United States (averaging 350–400 mg/d as opposed to 600–800 mg in the United States), and higher levels of dietary calcium are associated with a decreased risk of stroke.[86] In Western society, there is some evidence to suggest a negative effect on CHD. An RCT involving 1471 patients taking calcium or placebo for 5 years showed a significant increase in MI in the treatment group.[87] Findings of a meta-analysis of RCTs involving greater than 20,000 patients less than 40 years of age taking calcium supplements found higher rates of both MI and stroke in patients taking calcium supplements, with hazard ratios of stroke and MI in the range of 1.2 to 1.3.[88] The mechanism of a possible deleterious effect on vascular disease is unknown, although possibly related to calcium deposition in vascular walls.

VITAMIN K

Observational data suggest that both vitamin K intake and serum levels correlate with bone density.[89] Although there is currently no recommended level of vitamin K intake to optimize bone health, a number of calcium supplements now contain vitamin K, usually in a concentration of 40 μg/dose. By comparison, 100 g of romaine lettuce contains 100 μg,[90] and the RDA for vitamin K is 120 μg for men and 90 μg for women.

DEHYDROEPIANDROSTERONE

Dehydroepiandrosterone (DHEA) is an inactive precursor hormone formed in the adrenal cortex, and transformed into androgens and estrogens in peripheral tissues. Nearly all of it circulates as its water-soluble sulfate (DHEAS). After cholesterol, DHEAS is the second most abundant chemical in the bloodstream, with serum concentrations greater than 100 times that of testosterone in men, and greater than 1000 times that of estradiol in women. Concentrations peak in the third decade of life, and then gradually fall so that DHEAS concentrations in patients in their 70s are 20% to 30% of those found in young men and women.[91]

Many of the physiologic changes seen with aging, such as a decrease in muscle mass, increase in fat mass, and decrease in bone strength, are the same changes seen in individuals with sex hormone deficiency, and so it has been speculated that these physiologic changes seen in the elderly may be reversed or attenuated by DHEA supplementation. Low levels are also associated with cognitive decline, frailty, and increased mortality.[92] Small studies suggesting improvements in muscle mass and a sense of well-being from DHEA administration have encouraged its use.[93]

However, when DHEA has been subjected to RCTs, positive effects from have been modest, and not accompanied by an improved sense of well-being. In the DHEAge study, 280 elderly men and women in France were given DHEA 50 mg/d or placebo for 1 year with no effect on muscle strength or body composition.[94] In an RCT involving 144 men and women who received DHEA or placebo (some men also received testosterone) for 2 years, there was no improvement in muscle strength, endurance, or insulin sensitivity.[95] Women in this study who were treated with DHEA did have a lowering of their high-density lipoprotein cholesterol by 5 mg/dL. An RCT of 225 adults aged 55 to 85 showed no effect on cognitive function or well-being over 1 year,[96] similar to the findings of an earlier meta-analysis.[97] DHEA has not been shown to improve cognition in patients with AD.[98] Declining levels of DHEA are more likely a marker rather than a cause of frailty.[99] To date, trials have involved relatively small numbers of patients.

DHEA is available by prescription in Canada and Europe, but in the United States it is currently classified as a supplement, and so can be purchased over the counter. DHEA is a banned substance in the Olympics and international athletic competitions.

GINKGO BILOBA

Ginkgo biloba leaf extract contains a number of plant-produced hydrocarbons that may protect neurons from oxidative damage. A standardized ginkgo preparation, UGb761, has been used in most recent ginkgo trails at a dose of 120 mg twice daily. Data to support its use is often of low quality. In a 1998 meta-analysis of the effect of ginkgo in treating mild AD, of greater than 50 articles reviewed, only 4 RCTs met the reviewers' criteria for rigor, only 212 patients were included, and treatment duration was only 3 to 6 months.[100]

Ginkgo has been promoted as a memory enhancer; however, detailed neuropsychological testing failed to show any effect of 120 mg of ginkgo in 230 middle-aged and elderly men and women treated for 6 months in a 2002 study.[101] There were trends toward ginkgo having a protective effect on memory in a group of 118 patients enrolled in an RCT followed for 42 months; however, the study was underpowered to demonstrate a protective effect.[102] For patients who already have cognitive decline, a 2009 Cochrane review concluded that the evidence that ginkgo results in clinically significant benefit is "unreliable." [103]

The publicly funded Ginkgo Evaluation of Memory is the largest RCT of ginkgo and includes 3069 patients with normal cognition (n = 2587) or mild cognitive impairment (n = 482). G biloba at 120 mg twice a day for 5 years has not been effective in reducing either the incidence of dementia or AD,[104] nor has it shown any cognitive benefits, even with detailed testing.[105]

A second large, ongoing RCT of ginkgo in patients at risk for dementia is the GuidAge study, a pharmaceutical manufacturer-sponsored trial involving 2854 participants in France whose average age is 76 and who presented to their family physician with a memory complaint but who did not have AD. Although conversion to AD was not different between treatment and placebo groups, for patients enrolled for ≥4 years, there was a difference in AD incidence of statistical significance (1.6% vs 3%). These results were announced by the sponsoring pharmaceutical manufacturer, but have not appeared in a peer-reviewed publication.[106]

OMEGA-3 FATTY ACIDS

Omega-3 fatty acids (O3FA) are essential fatty acids found in fish, green leafy vegetables, walnuts, and a few oils such as canola, flaxseed, and soybean. Eicosapentaenoic acid and docosahexaenoic acid, both precursors of anti-inflammatory mediators, are the 2 most studied O3FAs, and have been studied primarily in the areas of preventing heart disease and dementia. O3FAs are unlikely to have a role in cancer prevention.[107]

Based on prospective studies demonstrating that fish and dietary O3FA consumption lower heart disease mortality, the American Heart Association recommends that everyone eat fish at least twice weekly, and also include in their diets oils high in O3FA. For patients with known CHD, the American Heart Association also recommends patients consume approximately 1 g of O3FA each day, preferably from fish.[108] To successfully ingest 1 g, many patients with CHD need to use supplements. One serving of salmon or sardines contains greater than 1 gram of O3FA, but most other commonly consumed fish contain less than half this amount. (Walnut and canola oil contain a little greater than 1 gram per tablespoon; flaxseed oil, almost 7 g).[109]

Observational studies of the effect of dietary O3FA consumption on cognitive decline have generally shown either small or inconsistent results,[110–112] and 302 elderly patients showed no cognitive benefits from 6 months of O3FA supplements in an RCT.[113] In 204 patients with mild AD treated with 2.3 g of O3FA, a small subset of 32 patients with very mild disease (Mini Mental State Examination score >27) showed a significant decrease in the rate of measured cognitive decline.[114] Most O3FA supplements list the dose as docosahexaenoic acid + eicosapentaenoic acid and contain approximately 900 mg and an extra 20 calories.

REFERENCES

1. Féart C, Samieri C, Rondeau V, et al. Adherence to a Mediterranean diet, cognitive decline, and risk of dementia. JAMA 2009;302:638–48.

44. Johansson M, Relton C, Ueland P, et al. Serum B vitamin levels and risk of lung cancer. JAMA 2010;303:2377–85.

45. Egging M, Bonaa K, Nygard O, et al. Cancer incidence and mortality after treatment with folic acid and vitamin B_{12}. JAMA 2009;302:2119–53.

46. Lindenbaum J, Healton E, Savage D, et al. Neuropsychiatric disorders caused by cobalmin deficiency in the absence of anemia or macrocytosis. N Engl J Med 1988;318:1720–8.

47. Brouwer I, Verhoef. Folic acid fortification: is masking of vitamin B12 deficiency what we should really worry about? Am J Clin Nutr 2007;86:897–8.

48. Andres E, Affenberger S, Vinzio S, et al. Food-cobalamin malabsorption in elderly patients: clinical manifestations and treatment. Am J Med 2005;118:1154–9.

49. de Jager J, Kooy A, Lehert P, et al. Long term treatment with metformin in patients with type 2 diabetes and risk of vitamin B-12 deficiency: randomized placebo controlled trial. BMJ 2010;340:c2181.

50. Elia M. Oral or parenteral therapy for B12 deficiency. Lancet 1998;352:1721–2.

51. Marks J. The safety of the vitamins: an overview. Int J Vitam Nutr Res Suppl 1989;30:12–20.

52. Holick M. Vitamin D deficiency. N Engl J Med 2007;357:266–81.

53. Heaney R, Davies K, Chen T, et al. Human serum 25-hydroxycholecalciferol response to extended oral dosing with cholecalciferol. Am J Clin Nutr 2003;77: 204–10.

54. Vitamin D and health. About Health Canada. Available at: www.hc-sc.gc.ca. Accessed October 12, 2010.

55. Davis C. Vitamin D and health in the 21st century: an update vitamin D and cancer: current dilemmas and future research needs. Am J Clin Nutr 2008;88:565S–9S.

56. Bischoff-Ferrari H, Giovannucci E, Willett W, et al. Estimation of optimal serum concentrations of 25-hydroxyvitamin D for multiple health outcomes. Am J Clin Nutr 2006;84:18–28.

57. Wortsman J, Matsuoka L, Chen T, et al. Decreased bioavailability of vitamin D in obesity. Am J Clin Nutr 2000;72:690–3.

58. Bischoff-Ferrari H, Willett W, Wong J, et al. Fracture prevention with vitamin D supplementation. JAMA 2005;293:2257–64.

59. Bischoff-Ferrari H, Willett W, Wong J, et al. Prevention of nonvertebral fractures with oral vitamin D and dose dependency. Arch Intern Med 2009;169:551–61.

60. Bischoff-Ferrari H, Dawson-Hughes B, Willett W, et al. Effect of vitamin D on falls. JAMA 2004;291:1999–2006.

61. Bischoff-Ferrari H, Dawson-Hughes B, Staehelin H, et al. Fall prevention with supplemental and active forms of Vitamin D. BMJ 2009;393:b3692.

62. Bischoff-Ferrari H, Dietrich T, Orav E, et al. Higher 25-hydroxyvitamin d concentration are associated with better lower-extremity function in both active and inactive persons aged ≥60y. Am J Clin Nutr 2004;80:752–8.

63. Gorham ED, Garland CF, Garland FC, et al. Optimal vitamin D status for colorectal cancer prevention: a quantitative meta analysis. Am J Prev Med 2007;32:210–6.

64. Bischoff-Ferrari H, Gioannucci W, Willett W, et al. Estimation of optimal serum concentrations of 25-hydroxyvitamin D for multiple health outcomes. Am J Clin Nutr 2006;84:18–28.

65. Wactawski-Weride J, Kotchen J, Anderson G, et al. Calcium plus Vitamin D supplementation and the risk of colorectal cancer. N Engl J Med 2006;354:684–96.

66. Lappe J, Travers-Gustafson D, Davies K, et al. Vitamin D and calcium supplementation roduces cancer risk; results of a randomized trial. Am J Clin Nutr 2007;85: 1586–91.

67. Hsai J, Heiss G, Ren H, et al. Cardiovascular disease in women, calcium/vitamin D supplementation and cardiovascular events. Circulation 2007;115:846–54.
68. Melamed ML, Michos ED, Post W, et al. 25-hydroxyl Vitamin D levels and the risk of mortality in the general population. Arch Intern Med 2008;168:1629–37.
69. Giovannucci E, Liu Y, Hollis B, et al. 25-hydroxyvitamin D and risk of myocardial infarction in men: a prospective study. Arch Intern Med 2008;168:1174–80.
70. Wang T, Pencina M, Booth S, et al. Vitamin D deficiency and risk of cardiovascular disease. Circulation 2008;117:503–11.
71. Freedman B, Wagenknecht L, Hairston K, et al. Vitamin D, adiposity, and calcified atherosclerotic plaque in African-Americans. J Clin Endocrinol Metab 2010;95: 1076–83.
72. Forman J, Giovannucci E, Holmes M, et al. Plasma 25-hydroxyvitamin D levels and risk of incident hypertension. Hypertension. 2007;49:1063–9.
73. Plotnikoff G, Quigley J. Prevalence of severe hypovitaminosis D in patients with persistent, nonspecific musculoskeletal pain. Mayo Clin Proc 2003;78:1463–70.
74. Autier P, Gandini S. Vitamin D supplementation and total mortality: a meta-analysis of randomized controlled trial. Arch Intern Med 2007;167:1730–7.
75. Vieth R. Why the optimal requirement for vitamin D3 is probably much higher than what is officially recommended for adults. J Steroid Biochem Mol Biol 2004;89–90: 575–9.
76. Jones G. Pharmacokinetics of vitamin D toxicity. Am J Clin Nutr 2008;88:582S–6S.
77. Trang H, Cole D, Rubin L, et al. Evidence that vitamin D_3 increases serum 25-hydroxyvitamin D more efficiently than does vitamin D_2. Am J Clin Nutr 1998;68: 854–8.
78. Trivedi D, Doll R, Khaw K. Effect of four monthly oral vitamin D3 (cholecalciferol) supplementation on fractures and mortality in men and women living in the community: randomized double blind controlled trial. BMJ 2003;326:469–72.
79. Sanders K, Stuart A, Williamson E, et al. Annual High-Dose Oral vitamin D and falls and fractures in older women: a randomized controlled trial. JAMA 2010; 303:1815–22.
80. Hunt C, Johnson L. Calcium requirements: new estimations for men and women by cross-sectional statistical analyses of calcium balance data from metabolic studies. Am J Clin Nutr 2007;86:1054–63.
81. Wu K, Willett WC, Fuchs CS, et al. Calcium intake and risk of colon cancer in women and men. J Natl Cancer Inst 2002;94:437–46.
82. Grau MV, Baron JA, Sandler RS, et al. Prolonged effect of calcium supplementation on risk of colorectal adenomas in a randomized trial. J Natl Cancer Inst 2007;99: 129–36.
83. Jackson RD, LaCroix AZ, Gass M, et al. Calcium plus vitamin D supplementation and the risk of fractures. N Engl J Med 2006;354:669–83.
84. Chan J, Stampfer M, Ma J, et al. Dairy products, calcium, and prostate cancer risk in the Physicians' Health Study. Am J Clin Nutr 2001;74:549–54.
85. Allen N, Key T, Appleby P, et al. Animal foods, protein, calcium and prostate cancer: the European prospective investigation into cancer and nutrition. Br J Cancer 2008;98:1574–81.
86. Umesawa M, Iso H, Date C, et al. Dietary intake of calcium in relation to mortality from cardiovascular disease. Stroke 2006;37:20–6.
87. Bolland M, Barber P, Doughty R, et al. Vascular events in healthy older women receiving calcium supplementation: randomized controlled trial. BMJ 2008;336: 262–6.

110. MacLean CH, Newberry SJ, Mojica WA, et al. Effects of omega-3 fatty acids on cognitive function with aging, dementia, and neurological diseases. Summary, evidence report/technology assessment: number 114 (AHRQ publication number 05-E011-1). February 2005. Rockville (MD): Agency for Healthcare Research And Quality. Available at: http://www.ahrq.gov/clinic/epcsums/o3cogsum.htm.

111. Devore E, Grodstein F, van Rooij F, et al. Dietary intake of fish and omega-3 fatty acids in relation to long-term dementia risk. Am J Clin Nutr 2009;91(1):170–6.

112. Kroger E, Verreault R, Carmichael PH, et al. Omega-3 fatty acids and risk of dementia: the Canadian Study of Health and Aging. Am J Clin Nutr 2009;90(1):184–92.

113. van de Rest O, Geleijnse JM, Kok FJ, et al. Effect of fish oil on cognitive performance in older subjects: a randomized, controlled trial. Neurology 2008;71(6):430–8.

114. Freund-Levi Y, Eriksdotter-Jönhagen M, Cederholm T, et al. Omega-3 fatty acid treatment in 174 patients with mild to moderate Alzheimer disease: OmegAD Study, a randomized double-blind trial. Arch Neurol 2006;63:1402–8.

Aging and Toxins

Asma B. Jafri, MD, MAcM[a,b,c]

KEYWORDS

- Toxins • Environmental health • Elderly • Geriatric • Aging
- Pollution

Aging is a complex phenomenon, with the interaction of genetics, disease, and environmental exposures. It is a challenge at times to separate the effects of the 3 on the process of aging. However, select epidemiologic studies and a review of aging processes shed light onto environmental toxins as a contributory factor to aging. A good example is the well-known effect of sun-related damage to the skin and premature aging with excessive exposure. Other toxins are ubiquitous in our environment and have shown harmful effects for the aging population in particular. This is owing to toxin damage to the various organ systems which are already in the process of decline owing to physiologic changes of aging. It is not surprising to note that some of the most dangerous toxins are prescription and over-the-counter (OTC) medications.

This articles addresses the common toxins in the everyday environment that have been shown to play a role in the aging process of healthy older adults and also the effect on diseases of the elderly. The goal is to help the reader discern the clinically important toxins and their effects on the health of the aging population. The reader should also develop an awareness of the toxins that may not be as common. The toxins whose effects have not been reliably documented with rigorous scientific studies are also discussed. Common toxins that are relevant to the elderly are discussed.

AIR POLLUTION

Air pollution has been linked to multiple health problems and is regularly reviewed by the US Environmental Protection Agency (EPA) for adverse health outcomes. Epidemiologic studies support its contributory role in organ dysfunction, particularly the pulmonary and cardiovascular system. The normal physiologic aging process puts the aging population at greater risk of disease and the added pathologic exposure to air pollution adds premature changes to the aging processes. Some of these changes

The author has nothing to disclose.
^a University of California, Riverside, California
^b University of California Los Angeles, Los Angeles, California
^c Department of Family Medicine, Riverside County Regional Medical Center, 26520 Cactus Avenue, Moreno Valley, CA 92555, USA
E-mail address: ajafri@co.riverside.ca.us

Clin Geriatr Med 27 (2011) 609–628
doi:10.1016/j.cger.2011.07.007
0749-0690/11/$ – see front matter © 2011 Published by Elsevier Inc.

geriatric.theclinics.com

are at a subclinical level for healthy aging population, but others are critical in their contribution to the burden of damage, dysfunction, or disease.

Air pollution is a general term that encompasses many environmental air-suspended gaseous, liquid, and particulate matter. The different components include carbon monoxide, nitrates, sulfur dioxide, ozone, lead, mercury, asbestos, tobacco smoke, and particulate matter. These pollutants are from vehicle emissions, tire fragmentation, road dust, power generation, industrial combustion, metal processing, construction and demolition activities, pollens, mold, forest fires, and residential wood burning. The effects of air pollution on the aging population vary according to the residential community and the neighboring polluting industries or activities.[1]

Some of the evidence from literature is reviewed to give a perspective of the clinical approach to addressing air pollution in the elderly population. It is clear from review of multiple original research and clinical review articles that air pollution is a significant contributor to morbidity and mortality in the elderly population. It is also prudent to examine the effects of indoor and outdoor air pollution separately because the exposure risk and type of pollutant materials are different. The homebound elderly spend almost all their time in the indoor environment and are at much higher risk of the effects of indoor air pollution compared with a younger and more mobile elderly population.

Outdoor Air Pollution

Air pollution is associated with cardiovascular deaths and hospital admissions, as has been demonstrated by numerous epidemiologic studies from around the world.[2] More than half the US population lives in areas where the air pollution exceeds the health standards set by the EPA.[3] The daily air pollution index is a good indicator of health risks associated with air pollution. Older adults are more vulnerable to the health risks of air pollution than their younger counterparts.[4] The EPA recommends for the elderly to avoid prolonged or heavy outdoor exertion at air pollution index of 101 to 150 (moderate). This is because of the unusual sensitivity of elderly lungs and cardiovascular system to the particulate matter and ozone. This is especially important in elderly with chronic obstructive pulmonary disease and preexisting heart disease, because they have mortality and morbidity related to air pollution. Ozone levels tend to be higher in the summer, especially in the high ultraviolet hours (10 AM–3 PM).

The underlying biochemical processes of air pollution have not been firmly established, but studies have shown the negative effects to involve the physiologic functions of various systems and cellular mechanisms. Studies have shown changes in heart rate variability,[5] electrocardiographic repolarization,[6] vascular function,[7] and C-reactive protein[5] with particulate air pollution. However, other studies did not find this association.[8] A Canadian prospective cohort study on the of effects of indoor, outdoor, and personal exposure to particulate air pollution showed that particulate matter was associated with increases in systolic and diastolic blood pressure, heart rate, and vascular endothelial growth factor.[9] Another retrospective cohort study of 1222 men from Greece who sought care at a hypertension clinic showed that air concentration of particulate matter was associated with increased blood pressure and aortic pulse pressure.[10] A third study from National Taiwan University showed that exposure to particulate matter and ozone was associated with increased blood pressure, blood lipids levels, fasting blood sugar level, and glycosylated hemoglobin levels.[11] Levels of glycosylated hemoglobin and apolipoprotein B are associated with oxidative stress and dysfunctional endothelium and play an important role in the pathogenesis of atherosclerosis. Another study from the University of California, Irvine, showed a positive association of systolic and diastolic blood and pressure ambulatory blood pressure with air pollution.[12] The strongest association was with organic carbon, which is reflective of the fossil fuel combustion (traffic-related air pollution).

Particles >10 um are usually trapped in the upper airways, and smaller ones may be deposited in the lining of the lower airways and alveoli. Pollution-generating smaller suspended particles are of major concern to the health of a person.

Schwartz[13] found a higher rate of out-of-hospital deaths compared with in-hospital deaths in looking at the relationship of airborne particulate matter exposure and daily deaths in 10 large US cities.[13] Dennekamp et al[14] from Australia showed an association between daily average air pollution particularly PM2.5 and out-of-hospital cardiac arrests. This study had 8434 outcome events over age 35. It has been suggested by another study that those who are already treated for coronary heart disease may be less susceptible to air pollution.[15] This is an interesting observation, and is counterintuitive to what we know about the effects of air pollution and effects on disease. This reduced susceptibility maybe be theoretically explained by the modulating effects of medications taken for coronary heart disease, particularly aspirin with its anti-inflammatory effects.

A major link of the effects of air pollution on cardiovascular disease is the effect of air pollution on the cardiac rhythm and the autonomic control of cardiac rhythm. The autonomic control of the heart is measured by heart rate variability. Liao et al[16] showed that elevated concentrations of PM2.5 are associated with lower heart rate variability. Lower heart rate variability has been related to sudden cardiac death and increased risk of developing coronary heart disease.[17,18]

It is prudent to appreciate the negative effect of air pollution, particularly particulate matter air pollution, on cardiovascular disease in the elderly. Persons with higher level exposures and persons with lung or cardiovascular disease are the most vulnerable populations. Particular attention should be paid to seniors who live in large, metropolitan areas with greater exposure to smoke, soot, and fossil fuel combustion. To avoid unnecessary pollutant exposure, seniors should be advised not to exercise outdoors when the air pollution index is >50. Exercise leads to increased deposition of particles in the lung tissues owing to increased ventilation. One study showed a 5-fold increase in total deposition of small particles in the lung tissues during moderate exercise.[19]

Indoor Air Pollution

Most elderly spend 80% to 90% of their day indoors, causing increased indoor air pollution exposure. Few studies have looked at the effect of indoor air pollution on chronic or preexisting diseases. Hopefully, we will have more information on this topic in the future with the focus on the elderly. For a detailed review of indoor air quality and various pollutants the reader is referred to the free downloadable PDF titled "An Introduction for Health Professional: Indoor Air Quality/US EPA."[20]

Indoor air pollution depends on the outdoor air pollution and on suspended particulate matter generated from indoor fixtures, cleaning, renovation and cooking. Ozone levels tend to be 10% to 80% lower than outdoor levels.[21]

Environmental tobacco smoke (ETS), nitrogen dioxide (NO_2), and respiratory suspended particles are the 3 major indoor air pollutants. An association between indoor respiratory suspended particles and worsening respiratory symptoms have been found in the few studies available.[22,23] NO_2 is produced by indoor burning natural gas, kerosene, and propane. NO_2 has been shown to cause lung damage at high concentrations and symptoms of irritation of the nose and eyes.[24] Two studies have shown increased respiratory symptoms and decreased lung function in adults (males and females) and using gas for cooking.[25] NO$_2$ levels of indoor NO$_2$ tend to be higher in the kitchen in the winter months.[26]

ETS

Cigarette smoking has been identified as a major risk factor for cancers of the oral cavity, esophagus, stomach, pancreas, larynx, lung, bladder, and kidney. It is associated with increased risk of ischemic heart disease, aortic aneurysm, chronic obstructive lung disease, stroke, pneumonia, cirrhosis, cancer of the liver, and acute myeloid leukemia.[27] We do not discuss the effects of first-hand cigarette smoking because it is beyond the scope of this article and warrants a separate discussion.

Secondhand smoke (SHS), also known as ETS, is the single major indoor air pollutant when a smoker is around. It has special implications in the aging population. Fortunately, most states have strict regulations for smoking in public places and institutional settings. Tobacco smoke has >4000 compounds, many of which are known carcinogens and irritants. The effects of tobacco smoke (home and occupational) on the incidence of lung cancer are well recognized.[28,29] Previous research has shown that even exposure to 1 secondhand cigarette smoke accelerates the progression of atherosclerosis.[30]

Indoor exposure to ETS is associated with respiratory symptoms and reduced lung function in adults.[31] The mortality from smoking-related diseases is more prominent among those older than age 60, owing to the prolonged exposure over the years and the latency in development of diseases. A secondhand smoker inhales nicotine, benzene, and tobacco smoke carcinogens. Cotinine, the principal metabolite of nicotine, is detected in secondhand smokers at almost the same rates as smokers. A 31-country study found that the median air levels of nicotine was 17 times higher in the homes where smoking took place compared with other homes.[32] The surgeon general has concluded that the evidence is sufficient to infer that exposure of nonsmokers to SHS causes an increased risk of lung cancers.[33] The risk for cardiovascular disease is increased in SHS, with an estimated 40,000 heart disease–related deaths each year in the United States.[34] The increased risk for heart disease seems to be owing to endothelial dysfunction, similar to that in active smokers. A study found that exposure to SHS was associated with increased levels of several markers of inflammation (white blood cells, C-reactive protein, homocystine, fibrinogen, and low-density lipoprotein cholesterol).[35]

A study in China found an association between SHS and stroke prevalence in women. The prevalence of stroke increased with the longer duration of exposure and the number of cigarettes smoked per day.[36]

A meta-analysis of 29 cross-sectional studies showed that cigarette smoking was associated with decreased bone mineral density and 41% increase in risk for hip fracture at age 70.[37] The adverse health risks for SHS can be found at www.surgeongeneral.gov/library/reports/index/html.

ALCOHOL

Alcohol is a unique health issue for the older person; there are reported health benefits of moderate consumption of alcohol, particularly red wine, and at the same time there are unique deleterious health effects for some cohorts of the elderly. The current National Institute on Alcohol Abuse and Alcoholism guidelines suggest that older adults limit alcohol intake to 1 drink per day for both genders. A drink is defined as 12 oz of beer, 5 oz of wine, or 1.5 oz of spirits. The prevalence of moderate alcohol use in 2000/2001, based on 3 national representative cross surveys, was 37.6% in elderly males compared with 32.3% in elderly females. The prevalence for heavy alcohol use was 10.1% in males compared with 2.2% in females.[38] Binge drinking was reported in 14% of men and in 3% of women >65 years old in 1 survey.[39]

Ethanol is a physiologically nonessential, energy (7 Kcal/g) molecule produced by fermentation of pyruvate from plants that have a high carbohydrate content. It does not require gastrointestinal (GI) digestion; therefore, the immediate effects are seen quickly. Approximately 2% of alcohol undergoes inactivation by gastric alcohol dehydrogenase (ADH). Adult men have greater ADH activity than women, so bioavailability of the same amount of alcohol consumed is greater in women. Older adults have decreased gastric ADH activity leading to increased bioavailability of alcohol consumed.[40] The remaining alcohol is metabolized by the hepatocyte ADH to acetaldehyde at a maximum rate of 15 g/h.[41] Alcohol is also metabolized by inducible microsomal ethanol oxidizing system. Other drugs and nutrients are metabolized by the microsomal ethanol oxidizing system, leading to drug interactiuons.[42] For the same amount of alcohol consumed, the elderly have higher blood alcohol levels than younger persons of the same body mass and gender.[43]

One of the challenges in the senior population is that the usual social and occupational markers for excess alcohol consumption (eg, driving under the influence, job problems, marital problems) are not there. Seniors maybe more exclusive in their social environment and may not drive. Physicians and other health care professionals may be the only personnel who have access to screen these individuals for immoderate alcohol intake. High-risk alcohol intake was more prevalent among persons 60 to 64 years of age, Caucasians, and have lower education.[44] Women may use alcohol more for self-medication and mood disorders, and are at higher risk for deleterious health effects of alcohol compared with men.[45,46]

The effects of moderate alcohol consumption, particularly red wine, on cardiovascular health are well-reported in literature.[47] There is evidence that all-cause mortality is reduced with mild to moderate alcohol consumption.[48] There is a U- or J-shaped relationship between alcohol intake and mortality in the elderly.[49] These beneficial effects are nullified when alcohol consumption is more than moderate.[50]

Heavy alcohol use is associated with dementia, cerebellar degeneration, and Wernicke-Korsakoff syndrome.[51] A systematic review showed that small amounts of alcohol may be protective against dementia and Alzheimer's disease, but not against vascular dementia.[52] The behavioral effects of alcohol are dose and time related. The effects of moderate alcohol (pleasure, stress reduction, and anxiolysis) are perceived as reinforcing. Moderate alcohol intake had both a diminution and positive effect on cognition.[53] A prospective cohort study showed that consumption of spirits in women was associated with a slightly increased risk of dementia, whereas wine was protective for dementia.[54] It is unclear whether the protective effects can be ascribed to alcohol or specific components, namely, polyphenols.

A population-based sample showed radiologic (magnetic resonance imaging) changes of brain white matter lesions and infarcts were lower in light-to-moderate intake of alcohol compared with abstention and heavy drinking.[55] Moderate intake of alcohol has also been reported to be associated with positive effects on bowl elimination, reduction in risk for osteoporosis, and reduced incidence of diabetes mellitus.[56]

ENVIRONMENTAL TEMPERATURE EXPOSURES

The aging population is particularly at risk for adverse effects of heat as well as extreme cold. This is because of the physiologic changes that occur with aging that impair the physiologic homostatic mechanisms inherent for survival.

Heat Exposure

Excessive ambient heat exposures may result in excess mortality in the elderly as 1 of the vulnerable populations.[57] In a previous analysis by the US Centers for Disease Control and Prevention, heat-related deaths have been based on underlying cause entered on the death certificates and have not included decedents for whom hyperthermia was listed as a contributing factor, but not the underlying cause. When the analysis included the deaths where hyperthermia was listed as a contributing or underlying cause the heat related deaths increased by 54%. From 1999 to 2003, a total of 3442 reported deaths resulted from exposure to extreme heat. Of those who died, 1363 (40%) were aged ≥65 years. The state with the highest death rate was Arizona (1.7 deaths per 100,000 population).[58]

Like cold, heat exposure risks are greatest for older people who are not used to living in hot weather, because they are generally not prepared to deal with a sudden or new onset of a heat wave or change in weather. Although comorbid illnesses and physiologic changes of aging with impaired homeostasis affect heat-related outcomes, lack of acclimatization and an inability to make environmental changes is also a contributing factor to increased morbidity and mortality related to heat exposure. The most important risk factor is lack of access to air conditioning. People living in apartment buildings, on upper floors, or in flat-roofed buildings are at increased risk.[59] A meta-analysis of 6 studies with 1065 deaths showed that confinement to a bed, not leaving home daily, psychiatric illness, and being unable to care for oneself were the main risk factors related to death. Working air conditioning, visiting cool environments, and increasing social contact were strongly associated with better outcomes.[60]

Excessive heat exposure can lead to hyperthermia or death.[58] Heat exhaustion and heat stroke are the most serious heat-related illnesses. Heat exhaustion is characterized by muscle cramps, fatigue, headache, nausea, vomiting, dizziness, and fainting. The skin is cool and moist with rapid heart rate and breathing. If untreated, heat exhaustion can progress to heat stroke. Heat stroke is a serious, life-threatening condition characterized by high body temperature (>103°F), red hot and dry skin, rapid and strong pulse, throbbing headache, dizziness, confusion, and unconsciousness. Symptoms can progress to encephalopathy, coagulopathy, and multiple organ failure.

Public health care professional and community-wide educational efforts are all important in local communities during a heat wave or unexpected sudden hot weather. The US Centers for Disease Control and Prevention website (www.cdc.gov) has excellent educational materials on heat stress in the elderly for the public and those who care for the elderly.

Cold Exposure and Hypothermia

As people age, their physiologic mechanisms for temperature regulation in extreme situations become less efficient. Subsequently, they are at increased risk of developing hypothermia when exposed to extreme cold. Moreover, the risk is magnified for elderly who have chronic disease and are taking multiple medications. Hypothermia can develop in the elderly from a variety of conditions, including exposure to cold environment, metabolic derangements, toxins, central nervous system dysfunction, and endocrinopathies. We focus on hypothermia owing to cold exposure because the other topics are beyond the scope of this article. The hypothermia owing to outdoor cold activities and sports is well-studied; protective techniques are applied well to prevent the incidence of hypothermia. Moreover, younger and healthier persons undertake such activities. However, most hypothermia deaths are from indoor exposure to extreme cold.

From 1999 to 2002, a total of 4607 death certificates in the United States had a hypothermia-related diagnosis listed as the underlying cause of death or nature of injury. Of the deceased, 49% were aged ≥65 and 83% of the deaths occurred between October and March.[61]

Hypothermia occurs when the core body temperature is <95°F. When a person is exposed to excessive cold and he/she cannot generate enough heat to keep the normal body temperature of 98.6°F, there is organ system and brain dysfunction. Signs and symptoms of hypothermia include lethargy, weakness, loss of coordination, confusion, or uncontrollable shivering. Data from the US Army suggest that males and females are equally susceptible; most civilians who die from hypothermia are males.[62]

The mechanisms for loss of body heat are through radiation, conduction, convection, evaporation, and respiration. Radiation heat is lost from the head and noninsulated parts of the body accounts for 50% of heat loss. Conduction is loss by direct contact and is important in immersion injuries; the conductivity of water is 3 times that of air. Convection heat loss occurs with the movement of fluid or gas. This is important in wind chill conditions where the warm air next to the skin is rapidly drawn away from the body. Evaporation and respiration is through water droplets and the heat loss owing to these mechanisms is worse in dry, cold, and windy weather.

The body homeostatic thermal mechanisms in cold environments are activated utilizing heat production and heat conservation. Heat production is achieved with shivering and nonshivering thermogenesis via increased epinephrine and thyroxine. Heat conservation is achieved by peripheral vasoconstriction. The systems of homeostasis are overwhelmed when the body is exposed to extreme cold for a prolonged period of time with depleted metabolic stores of glycogen and other substrates, resulting in an acidotic tissue environment. Hypothermia is classified as mild, moderate, or severe (**Table 1**).

The elderly are at risk for hypothermia when they do not have adequate heating arrangements in cold weather. The subtle symptoms of mild hypothermia may not be perceived as significant and continued exposure may lead to moderate or severe hypothermia, where the elderly may not have the mental clarity to protect themselves from further exposure or seek help.

The pathologic and clinical findings of hypothermia occur along a continuum. The elderly with mild hypothermia may have shivering, tachycardia, peripheral vasoconstriction (cold hands and feet), apathy, and impaired judgment. Moderate

Table 1	
Hypothermia	
Degree of Hypothermia	**Temperature, °C (°F)**
Mild	M32–35C (90–95)
Moderate	28–32C (82–90)
Severe	<28 (<82)

hypothermia, which heralds a poor outcome, has decreased heart rate, cessation of shivering, atrial dysrhythmias, decreased level of consciousness, decreased rate of respiration, and J wave (Osborne) on an electrocardiogram. Severe hypothermia is characterized by coma, pulmonary edema, apnea, ventricular fibrillation asystole, and death.

It is important for physicians to use special low-temperature thermometers or rectal thermistor probes when the regular thermometer reads <95°F because regular thermometers only read only down to 94°F.

When an elderly person is brought for emergency management, any wet clothing should be removed and replaced with blankets for insulation. Excessive movement or nasogastric tube placement should be avoided, because as these have been shown to precipitate ventricular fibrillation. Aggressive resuscitation with warmed fluids and warmed humidified oxygen should be undertaken. Active external rewarming (warm blankets, etc) has the complication of core temperature afterdrop when the cold peripheral blood rapidly returns to the heart. This complication can be avoided by using minimally invasive core rewarming before active external rewarming. The American Heart Association recommends treating ventricular fibrillation with defibrillation. If initially unsuccessful, withhold intravenous medications until the patient is warmed to 30°C (86°F). Asystole even for 2 hours does not represent irreversible cardiac compromise and attempts at resuscitation should continue until rewarming efforts achieve a core temperature of 30°C.[63] Active core rewarming can be done with extracorporal blood warming accomplished by cardiopulmonary bypass, arteriovenous rewarming, venovenous rewarming, or hemodialysis. These techniques are very effective at raising the core body temperature by 1°C to 3°C every 3 to 5 minutes. Immediate cardiopulmonary bypass rewarming is recommended for patients in ventricular fibrillation with core temperature <30°C.[64]

The elderly are high risk for developing hypothermia because of impaired thermoregulatory mechanisms; they may disregard the subtle symptoms and signs of early hypothermia and may not be able to make behavioral or environmental adjustments to protect themselves. Hence, community-wide interventions should target the elderly for public safety efforts in extreme cold climatic conditions.

PRESCRIPTION DRUGS

Prescription drugs are used by the elderly disproportionately compared with the rest of the population. Elderly account for 13% of the population but use >30% of prescribed drugs.[65] This is owing to a higher incidence of chronic diseases like arthritis, cardiovascular disease, diabetes, hypertension, dementia, and cancer. The use of different medications simultaneously puts the elderly at increased risk for drug–drug interactions, which results in more hospitalizations and in increased length of the hospital stay.[66] Changes in the biologic mechanisms that affect drug metabolism are briefly reviewed. There are 2 basic pharmacotherapeutic principles that account for better understanding of drug handling by the body: Pharmacokinetics and pharmacodynamics.[67]

The effects of nonsteroidal anti-inflammatory drugs (NSAIDs) on the GI tract are well known. NSAIDs inhibits prostaglandin synthesis in the stomach, leading to a loss of the protective mechanisms of the stomach against the corrosive effect of stomach acid. The adverse GI effects include GI bleeding, which is estimated to account for the 15th most common cause of death in the United States.[68] NSAIDs may lead to asymptomatic GI bleeding in the elderly. NSAIDs are on the BEERS criteria of drugs to avoid in the elderly.[69] NSAIDs also cause renal toxicity secondary to acute interstitial nephritis and to the blocking of the vasodilatory effects of prostaglandins on the efferent arterioles of the glomerulus. The elderly may have decreased creatinine clearance with normal serum creatinine levels. These persons may be prescribed NSAIDs in the usual dose with further progression of their renal impairment.

Benzodiazepines are a class of drugs with significant adverse effects in the elderly. All benzodiazepines are metabolized in the liver. The hepatic oxidation metabolism of drugs is decreased in the elderly. Benzodiazepines that are metabolized with oxidation should be avoided in the elderly. These include alprazolam, clonazepam, diazepam, midazolam, and triazolam. However, hepatic glucuronidation is not effected with aging. Lorazepam, oxazepam, and temazepam are the preferred benzodiazepines in the elderly because they are metabolized by glucuronidation. Shorter half-life benzodiazepines are preferred in the elderly. Old age has been reported to have increased intrinsic sensitivity to benzodiazepines.[70]

Coumadin has multiple drug–nutrient, drug–drug, and drug–disease interactions that can cause serious adverse effects. Advanced age is an independent risk factor for anticoagulation-induced hemorrhage. Coumadin has a narrow therapeutic window and a wide variability in dose response across individuals. It requires close monitoring of the International Normalized Ratio when it is started, dose adjustment is made, or a new drug is co-administered. Approximately 99% of coumadin is bound to plasma proteins and is metabolized through the CYP2C9 system. Drugs concomitantly used that are metabolized by the same enzyme in the liver or drugs that displace its protein-bound state may affect the bioavailability of the drug.[71] The drug's risk of bleeding is increased when it is used concomitantly with NSAIDs, aspirin, or macrolide antibiotics.[72]

OTC MEDICATIONS

There are 400,000 OTC medications available in the United States.[73] The elderly are extremely sensitive to adverse and toxic effects of OTC medications because of the physiologic changes that occur with aging. Older adults generally self-treat using OTC medications. They comprise 13% of the population, but accounts for 40% of purchase of OTC medications. Few elderly read the product label or leaflet information.[74] According to 1 study, 80.4% of chronically ill elderly were taking OTC.[75]

Of older adults presenting to emergency departments, 29% were taking potentially inappropriate medications with potential adverse drug effects.[76] Also worth noting is that in this study 16% of all medications prescribed in the emergency department were potentially inappropriate medications. A study showed that 83% of patients with moderate chronic renal insufficiency and 68% of patients with severe chronic renal insufficiency were using ≥1 OTC medication.[77] Patients with chronic renal insufficiency are greatest risk for severe adverse drug reactions with the inappropriate use of OTC medications because most are taking several prescribed medications.

The use of laxative medications is a particular problem in the elderly. They use laxatives inappropriately with the development of laxative tolerance and adverse effects.[78] There is a case report of laxative-induced rhabdomyolysis with the use of lactulose and sorbitol syrup.[79] Physicians are in a perfect position to educate patients on the safe and appropriate use of OTC medications depending on risks and contraindications in individual patients. A medicine cabinet history should be taken on all elderly patients.[80]

HERBAL MEDICATIONS

Herbal medications are plant products. They were designated as dietary supplements by the 1994 Drug Safety and Health Education Act. The use of herbal medications has increased in the United States over the last 2 decades. The use of dietary supplements increased from 14% in 1998 and 1999 to 18.8% in 2002. Use did not change among younger subjects, but doubled in persons older than age 65.[81]

A study done on the US–Mexican border showed that 255 of the survey participants had used an herbal supplement in the preceding 12 months.[82] Half of the adult participants in this study were at risk for potential drug–drug interactions and one third were at risk for potential drug–herbal interactions. There is no oversight on the content, safety, or efficacy of herbal medications. No animal testing is required before human trials and approval from the US Food and Drug Administration is not required. A new amendment to the Drug Safety and Health Education Act requires reporting of adverse effects to the US Food and Drug Administration.

The elderly may resort to using herbals owing to concerns of side effects with conventional medications. There are multiple drug–herb–disease interactions that should be avoided in elderly persons who are using multiple medications along with herbal products. Physicians should educate patients about concerns related to use of herbal medications, especially in those with chronic medical conditions and who are taking multiple medications. Patients are not as likely to disclose the use of herbal medications to their doctor, so physicians should put extra effort into obtaining this information.[83]

Ginseng abuse may cause hypertension, behavioral problems, and diarrhea.[84] When used with coumadin, it can reduce prothrombin time. A contaminant in ginseng called germanium can cause nephrotoxicity by damaging the cells of the ascending limb of the loop of Henle, thereby diminishing the responsiveness of loop diuretics (furosemide [Lasix, Sanofi-Aventis, Bridgewater, NJ]).[85]

Garlic inhibits platelet aggregation, so its use should be stopped 10 days before elective surgery.[86] Grapefruit juice is a strong inhibitor of CYP3A4 enzyme and increases the levels of CYP3A4 substrate drugs. Grapefruit juice may increase the risk of breast cancer by inhibiting estrogen metabolism in postmenopausal women taking estrogens.[87] Aconite is toxic and even contact with its leaves can cause bradycardia, hypotension, and fatal ventricular arrhythmias.[88] Black Cohosh is being used for the relief of postmenopausal symptoms, but has not been shown to be effective.[89] It can cause an increase in substrate drugs for CYP3A4 enzyme and can cause hepatotoxicity.[90]

Several herbal medications pose a serious risk of toxicity for the elderly population. Physicians should routinely review herbal medications used by their elderly patients and counsel patients on the risks and benefits based on the available scientific evidence.

DRINKING WATER

Drinking water in the United States is regulated by the Office of Ground Water and Drinking Water, which oversees the implementation of the Safe Drinking Water Act, the national law safeguarding tap water in America.[91] It protects ground water, and ensures safe drinking water Under the Safe Drinking Water Act. The EPA sets legal limits on the levels of certain contaminants in drinking water. The legal limits reflect both the level that protects human health and the level that water systems can achieve using the best available technology. Beside prescribing these legal limits, EPA rules set water-testing schedules and methods that water companies must follow. The rules also list acceptable techniques for treating contaminated water. The Safe Drinking Water Act gives individual states the opportunity to set and enforce their own drinking water standards if the standards are at least as strong as EPA's national standards. Most states and territories directly oversee the water systems within their

Box 1
Chemicals that are regulated by the EPA in drinking water
Aldrin and dieldrin
Boron
Dacthal and its degradates
1,1,-dichloro-2,2,-bis(p-chlorophenyl)ethylene (DDE)
1,3 dichloropropene
S-Ethyl dipropylthiocarbamate.
Fonofos
Hexachlorobutadiene
Manganese
Metribuzin
Naphthalene
Terbacil
1,1,2,2-Tetrachloroethane
Brominated trihalomethanes

borders.[91] There are approximately 50 chemicals and 10 microbial agents that are regulated by the EPA in drinking water (**Boxes 1** and **2**).

According to the EPA, the United States has 1 of the safest water supplies in the world. Advisory and scientific committees give regular reports to the EPA about potential or health risk contaminants that are not regulated. The process is extensive and takes a long time before a contaminant is added to the regulated list. The EPA publishes a Contaminant Candidate List every 5 years. Contaminants on the list are known or anticipated to occur in public water systems. The most current Contaminant Candidate List was published in October 2009 and contains 104 chemicals and 12 microbiologic contaminants. It contains a wide variety of industrial chemicals and a long list of pesticides. Approximately 10% to 15% of the population in the United States has private water supply that is unregulated. Private water testing organizations are available to test water for homeowners for a cost.

Using bottled water for drinking is a new trend in developed and developing countries. There is no evidence for the benefit of bottled water, except in natural

Box 2
Microbial agents regulated by the EPA in drinking water
Aeromonas
Cryptosporidium
Legionella
Giardia
Bacteria

disaster or emergency situations, when tap water may be contaminated. Better taste, which is touted as the reason for bottled water consumption, has not been supported by rigorous scientific evidence. Taste varies from faucet to faucet because water has to travel from a community supply source to a household.

Bottled water companies are known to use tap water. They are not required to disclose the source of the water on the label. The National Resources Defense Council reports that 25% to 30% of bottled water sold in the United States is tap water, which may or may not be treated.[92] A 1999 report found that some bottled water contains bacterial contaminants, organic chemicals, or inorganic contaminants.[93]

A 5-month inquiry in 2008 by the Associated Press documented the presence of a large number of pharmaceutical compounds in drinking water sources.[94] Chemicals from plastic bottles may be released into the water when bottles are stored in heat for prolonged periods of time. These chemicals include polycarbonate, bisphenol A (estrogen-like effect), vinyl chloride (known carcinogen), and diethyl adulate. There is also concern for bacterial growth after 48 hours of drinking from a bottle.[95]

Chlorine has been used since 1908 to disinfect tap water supplies in the United States. This is a confusing statement. Research studies have shown increased incidence of cancer in association with exposure to disinfection byproducts.[96] The World Health Organization International Agency for Research on Cancer noted methodologic limitations in the various studies that an association between chlorination and cancer. It stated that there is "inadequate evidence for the carcinogenicity of chlorinated drinking water in humans."[97]

There have been concerns about the arsenic, lead, nitrate, copper, and radionuclide levels in drinking water. Arsenic is found in the soil and enters the ground water supplies through erosion. It has been associated with increased risk for bladder, kidney, skin, and lung cancers. There is also possible increased risk for cardiovascular diseases and diabetes mellitus.[98] All of these diseases are more common in the elderly and any additional risk of arsenic exposure should be avoided.

Lead is a concern for older water systems, where lead-based plumbing may have been used. Symptoms of lead toxicity may be very subtle with mild cognitive changes, and physicians should maintain a high index of suspicion. A good history of house living environment and water supply may lead to testing of drinking water and a blood lead level.

Nitrates are not as big a concern for elderly as they are for young infants who can develop methemoglobinemia. The EPA has set the maximal contaminant levels at 10 mg/L. A potential risk for nitrates in food and water has been reported. Nitrates are reduced to nitrites, which interact with gut amines to form nitrosamine, a carcinogen. The gut bacteria provide the amines for the conversion to nitrosamine. The elderly, owing to achlorhydria, have bacterial overgrowth, which may promote increases in nitrosamine levels in the body. Nitrates are removed from the water by reverse osmosis, distillation, and ion exchange.[99]

Copper maximal contaminant levels are set at 1.3 mg/L by the EPA. Copper contamination occurs in well water from ground minerals or from plumbing. Water softeners actually increase copper levels in water. With hard water, the calcium and magnesium corrosive layer covers the copper pipes. This layer does not exist in soft water. Copper, when ingested above the maximal contaminant levels, can cause nausea, vomiting, and diarrhea. Persons with Wilson's disease and carriers of the gone for Wilson's disease are at risk for copper toxicity even with slightly higher levels of copper in the water.[100]

Well water should be tested annually for contaminant levels to ensure safe water for drinking. The US Centers for Disease Control and Prevention recommends running water (flushing) for 15 seconds anytime the faucet has not been used for ≥6 hours.[101]

Radionuclides are not as much a concern in the general population and the elderly. Most drinking water has low levels of radioactive contaminants, most of which are naturally occurring. At higher levels, long-term exposure to radionuclides in drinking water may cause cancer. It remains to be seen whether radionuclides from the radiologic and nuclear industries will cause an increase in the levels of radionuclides in drinking water.

RADIATION

The population is exposed to background non-ionizing and ionizing radiation (IR) on a daily basis. Non-ionizing radiation consists of sound waves, visible light, and microwaves. IR has a very high frequency and very short wavelength. IR most commonly comes in the form of gamma rays, x-rays, alpha particles, beta particles, and neutrons.[102]

IR has extremely high energy that strips electrons off atoms and at higher levels can even break up the nucleus. Ionization (the process of stripping electrons off atoms) releases high energy into the surrounding material that is able to disrupt the bonds between 2 carbon atoms. Radiation damages the molecules that regulate vital cell processes (eg, DNA and RNA) in living tissues. When damaged by radiation, cells repair the damage successfully, mutate during the repair process increasing the risk for cancer transformation, or suffer irreparable damage and die.[103]

A 1987 National Council on Radiation Protection and Measurement study found that 82% of IR exposure was from natural background radiation and 18% from man-made sources. Natural IR comes from radon, cosmic rays, terrestrial sources, and "internal" emissions.[103] Average annual natural background exposure in the United States is slightly higher (3.0 mSv) than the international average (2.4 mSv), in part because of higher average radon levels in the United States.[103] Man-made IR exposure was broken down to the following sources: Medical x-rays (58%), nuclear medicine (21%), consumer products (16%), occupational (2%), fallout (2%), and the nuclear fuel cycle (1%).

The health effects of radiation exposure vary by the dose received. Recent research in mice shows that low-dose radiation (10 cGy) induced genes not affected by high-dose radiation (2 Gy).[104] High does of radiation can result in burns and radiation sickness, which takes the form of nausea, weakness, hair loss, skin burns, and diminished organ function, and can lead to premature aging and death. A clinician is more likely to encounter and individual who is suffering from the effects of low-dose, low linear energy transfer.

The health effects of radiation include cardiovascular disease (coronary artery disease, stroke, and peripheral vascular disease) and hypertension.[105,106] There was a dose-related effect of radiation on heart disease mortality and incidence of hypertension.[107–109]

Cancer is the most widely known health effect of radiation exposure. The Board on Radiation Effects Research states that "the long latent period between radiation exposure and cancer development together with the multistage nature of tumorigenesis make it difficult to distinguish radiation-induced changes from those alterations that occur once the process has been initiated. Radiation-induced cancers do not appear to be unique or specifically identifiable."[110] The risk for cancer depends on the type of cancer, the dose and quality of the radiation, the dose rate, exposure to other carcinogens such as tobacco, and the age, gender, and other characteristics of the

29. Brown KG. Lung cancer and environmental tobacco smoke: occupational risk to nonsmokers. Environ Health Perspect 1999;107(Suppl 6):885–90.

30. American Heart Association. Air pollution, heart disease and stroke. 2010. Available at: http://www.americanheart.org/presenter.jhtml?identifier=4419. Accessed November 2010.

31. Hersoug LG, Husemoen LL, Sigsgaard T, et al. Indoor exposure to environmental cigarette smoke, but not other inhaled particulates associates with respiratory symptoms and diminished lung function in adults. Respirology 2010;15:993–1000.

32. Wipfli H, Avila-Tang E, Navas-Acien A, et al. Secondhand smoke exposure among women and children: evidence from 31 countries. Am J Public Health 2008;98:672–9.

33. US Department of Health and Human Services. The health consequences of involuntary exposure to tobacco smoke: A report of the surgeon general. 2006. Available at: http://www.surgeongeneral.gov/library/secondhandsmoke/report/. Accessed November 2010.

34. Glantz SA, Parmley WW. Passive smoking and heart disease. Mechanisms and risk. JAMA 1995;273:1047–53.

35. Panagiotakos DB, Pitsavos C, Chrysohoou C, et al. Effect of exposure to secondhand smoke on markers of inflammation: the ATTICA study. Am J Med 2004;116:145–50.

36. Zhang X, Shu XO, Yang G, et al. Association of passive smoking by husbands with prevalence of stroke among Chinese women nonsmokers. Am J Epidemiol 2005;161:213–8.

37. Jenkins MR, Denison AV. Smoking status as a predictor of hip fracture risk in postmenopausal women of northwest Texas. Prev Chronic Dis 2008;5:A09.

38. Breslow RA, Faden VB, Smothers B. Alcohol consumption by elderly Americans. J Stud Alcohol 2003;64:884–92.

39. Blazer DG, Wu LT. The epidemiology of substance use and disorders among middle aged and elderly community adults: national survey on drug use and health. Am J Geriatr Psychiatry 2009;17:237–45.

40. Pozzato G, Moretti M, Franzin F, et al. Ethanol metabolism and aging: the role of "first pass metabolism" and gastric alcohol dehydrogenase activity. J Gerontol A Biol Sci Med Sci 1995;50:B135–41.

41. Goodsell DS. The molecular perspective: alcohol. Oncologist 2006;11:1045–6.

42. Lieber CS. Relationships between nutrition, alcohol use, and liver disease. Alcohol Res Health 2003;27:220–31.

43. Lullmann H. Color atlas of pharmacology. 2nd edition. Stuttgart: Thieme; 2000.

44. Barnes AJ, Moore AA, Xu H, et al. Prevalence and correlates of at-risk drinking among older adults: the project SHARE study. J Gen Intern Med 2010;25:840–6.

45. Epstein EE, Fischer-Elber K, Al-Otaiba Z. Women, aging, and alcohol use disorders. J Women Aging 2007;19:31–48.

46. Brady KT, Randall CL. Gender differences in substance use disorders. Psychiatr Clin North Am 1999;22:241–52.

47. Goldberg IJ, Mosca L, Piano MR, et al. AHA science advisory: wine and your heart: a science advisory for healthcare professionals from the Nutrition Committee, Council on Epidemiology and Prevention, and Council on Cardiovascular Nursing of the American Heart Association. Circulation 2001;103:472–5.

48. Paganini-Hill A, Kawas CH, Corrada MM. Type of alcohol consumed, changes in intake over time and mortality: the Leisure World Cohort Study. Age Ageing 2007;36:203–9.

49. Gunzerath L, Faden V, Zakhari S, Warren K. National Institute on Alcohol Abuse and Alcoholism report on moderate drinking. Alcohol Clin Exp Res 2004;28:829–47.
50. Snow WM, Murray R, Ekuma O, et al. Alcohol use and cardiovascular health outcomes: a comparison across age and gender in the Winnipeg Health and Drinking Survey Cohort. Age Ageing 2009;38:206–12.
51. Anttila T, Helkala EL, Viitanen M, et al. Alcohol drinking in middle age and subsequent risk of mild cognitive impairment and dementia in old age: a prospective population based study. BMJ 2004;329:539.
52. Peters R, Peters J, Warner J, et al. Alcohol, dementia and cognitive decline in the elderly: a systematic review. Age Ageing 2008;37:505–12.
53. Eckardt MJ, File SE, Gessa GL, et al. Effects of moderate alcohol consumption on the central nervous system. Alcohol Clin Exp Res 1998;22:998–1040.
54. Mehlig K, Skoog I, Guo X, et al. Alcoholic beverages and incidence of dementia: 34-year follow-up of the prospective population study of women in Goteborg. Am J Epidemiol 2008;167:684–91.
55. den Heijer T, Vermeer SE, van Dijk EJ, et al. Alcohol intake in relation to brain magnetic resonance imaging findings in older persons without dementia. Am J Clin Nutr 2004;80:992–7.
56. Djousse L, Biggs ML, Mukamal KJ, et al. Alcohol consumption and type 2 diabetes among older adults: the Cardiovascular Health Study. Obesity (Silver Spring) 2007; 15:1758–65.
57. Basu R, Samet JM. Relation between elevated ambient temperature and mortality: a review of the epidemiologic evidence. Epidemiol Rev 2002;24:190–202.
58. Heat-related deaths—United States, 1999–2003. MMWR Morb Mortal Wkly Rep 2006;55:796–8.
59. Blum LN, Bresolin LB, Williams MA. From the AMA Council on Scientific Affairs. Heat-related illness during extreme weather emergencies. JAMA 1998;279:1514.
60. Bouchama A, Dehbi M, Mohamed G, et al. Prognostic factors in heat wave related deaths: a meta-analysis. Arch Intern Med 2007;167:2170–6.
61. Hypothermia-related deaths—United States, 1999–2002 and 2005. MMWR Morb Mortal Wkly Rep 2006;55:282–4.
62. Degroot DW, Kenney WL. Impaired defense of core temperature in aged humans during mild cold stress. Am J Physiol Regul Integr Comp Physiol 2007;292:R103–8.
63. Southwick FS, Dalglish PH Jr. Recovery after prolonged asystolic cardiac arrest in profound hypothermia. A case report and literature review. JAMA 1980;243:1250–3.
64. Splittgerber FH, Talbert JG, Sweezer WP, Wilson RF. Partial cardiopulmonary bypass for core rewarming in profound accidental hypothermia. Am Surg 1986;52:407–12.
65. Wilhelm M. The use of OTC medication in older adults. US Pharm 2009;34:44–7.
66. Bellomo A, Mancinella M, Iori A, et al. [Adverse drug reactions: a common cause of hospitalization of the elderly]. Recent Prog Med 2009;100:17–9.
67. Corsonello A, Pedone C, Incalzi RA. Age-related pharmacokinetic and pharmaco-dynamic changes and related risk of adverse drug reactions. Curr Med Chem 2010;17:571–84.
68. Prybys KM. Deadly drug interactions in emergency medicine. Emerg Med Clin North Am 2004;22:845–63.
69. Fick DM, Cooper JW, Wade WE, et al. Updating the Beers criteria for potentially inappropriate medication use in older adults: results of a US consensus panel of experts. Arch Intern Med 2003;163:2716–24.

70. Greenblatt DJ, Harmatz JS, Shader RI. Clinical pharmacokinetics of anxiolytics and hypnotics in the elderly. Therapeutic considerations (Part I). Clin Pharmacokinet 1991;21:165–77.
71. Jacobs LG. Warfarin pharmacology, clinical management, and evaluation of hemorrhagic risk for the elderly. Cardiol Clin 2008;26:157–67.
72. Snaith A, Pugh L, Simpson CR, et al. The potential for interaction between warfarin and coprescribed medication: a retrospective study in primary care. Am J Cardiovasc Drugs 2008;8:207–12.
73. Bednar B. OTC medication-induced nephrotoxicity in the elderly and CKD patient. Nephrol News Issues 2009;23:36.
74. Batty GM, Oborne CA, Swift CG, et al. The use of over-the-counter medication by elderly medical in-patients. Postgrad Med J 1997;73:720–2.
75. Guirguis K. The use of nonprescription medicines among elderly patients with chronic illness and their need for pharmacist interventions. Consult Pharm 2010;25:433–9.
76. Nixdorff N, Hustey FM, Brady AK, et al. Potentially inappropriate medications and adverse drug effects in elders in the ED. Am J Emerg Med 2008;26:697–700.
77. Laliberte MC, Normandeau M, Lord A, et al. Use of over-the-counter medications and natural products in patients with moderate and severe chronic renal insufficiency. Am J Kidney Dis 2007;49:245–56.
78. Kosseifi S, Nassour D, Byrd RP Jr, et al. Fatal iatrogenic hyperphosphatemia. J KY Med Assoc 2008;106:431–4.
79. Merante A, Gareri P, Marigliano NM, et al. Laxative-induced rhabdomyolysis. Clin Interv Aging 2010;5:71–3.
80. Vacas Rodilla E, Castella Daga I, et al. [Self-medication and the elderly. The reality of the home medicine cabinet]. Aten Primaria 2009;41:269–74.
81. Kelly JP, Kaufman DW, Kelley K, et al. Recent trends in use of herbal and other natural products. Arch Intern Med 2005;165:281–6.
82. Loya AM, Gonzalez-Stuart A, Rivera JO. Prevalence of polypharmacy, polyherbacy, nutritional supplement use and potential product interactions among older adults living on the United States-Mexico border: a descriptive, questionnaire-based study. Drugs Aging 2009;26:423–36.
83. Eisenberg DM, Davis RB, Ettner SL, et al. Trends in alternative medicine use in the United States, 1990–1997: results of a follow-up national survey. JAMA 1998;280:1569–75.
84. Siegel RK. Ginseng abuse syndrome. Problems with the panacea. JAMA 1979;241:1614–5.
85. Becker BN, Greene J, Evanson J, et al. Ginseng-induced diuretic resistance. JAMA 1996;276:606–7.
86. Gardner CD, Lawson LD, Block E, et al. Effect of raw garlic vs commercial garlic supplements on plasma lipid concentrations in adults with moderate hypercholesterolemia: a randomized clinical trial. Arch Intern Med 2007;167:346–53.
87. Monroe KR, Murphy SP, Kolonel LN, et al. Prospective study of grapefruit intake and risk of breast cancer in postmenopausal women: the Multiethnic Cohort Study. Br J Cancer 2007;97:440–5.
88. Smith SW, Shah RR, Hunt JL, et al. Bidirectional ventricular tachycardia resulting from herbal aconite poisoning. Ann Emerg Med 2005;45:100–1.
89. Pockaj BA, Gallagher JG, Loprinzi CL, et al. Phase III double-blind, randomized, placebo controlled crossover trial of black cohosh in the management of hot flashes: NCCTG Trial N01CC1. J Clin Oncol 2006;24:2836–41.

90. Chow EC, Teo M, Ring JA, et al. Liver failure associated with the use of black cohosh for menopausal symptoms. Med J Aust 2008;188:420–2.
91. US Environmental Protection Agency. Office of Water. 2010. Available at: http://water.epa.gov/. Accessed November 2010.
92. National Resources Defense Council. What's on Tap? Grading Drinking Water in U.S. Cities. New York: National Resources Defense Council; 2003.
93. Chalupka S. Tainted water on tap: what to tell patients about preventing illness from drinking water. Am J Nurs 2005;105:40–52.
94. Associated Press. An AP investigation: pharmaceuticals found in drinking water. 2008. Available at: http://hosted.ap.org/specials/interactives/pharmawater_site/. Accessed November 2010.
95. Raj SD. Bottled water: how safe is it? Water Environ Res 2005;77:3013–8.
96. Morris RD, Audet AM, Angelillo IF, et al. Chlorination, chlorination by-products, and cancer: a meta-analysis. Am J Public Health 1992;82:955–63.
97. International Agency for Research on Cancer. Chlorinated drinking-water; chlorination by-products; some other halogenated compounds; cobalt and cobalt compounds, volume 52. Lyon: International Agency for Research on Cancer; 1991.
98. Napier GL, Kodner CM. Health risks and benefits of bottled water. Prim Care 2008;35:789–802.
99. US Centers for Disease Control and Prevention. Nitrate and Drinking Water from Private Wells. 2009. available at: http://www.cdc.gov/healthywater/drinking/private/wells/disease/nitrate.html. Accessed November 2010.
100. National Research Council (US), Committee on Copper in Drinking Water. Copper in drinking water. Washington (DC): National Academy Press; 2000.
101. US Centers for Disease Control and Prevention. Copper and drinking water from private wells. 2010. Available at: http://www.cdc.gov/healthywater/drinking/private/wells/disease/copper.html. Accessed November 2010.
102. US Environmental Protection Agency. Radiation protection: understanding radiation. 2010. Available at: http://www.epa.gov/rpdweb00/understand/index.html. Accessed November 2010.
103. US National Research Council, Committee to Assess Health Risks from Exposure to Low Level of Ionizing Radiation. Executive Summary. Health risks from exposure to low levels of ionizing radiation: BEIR VII Phase 2. Washington (DC): National Academies Press; 2006.
104. Lowe XR, Bhattacharya S, Marchetti F, et al. Early brain response to low-dose radiation exposure involves molecular networks and pathways associated with cognitive functions, advanced aging and Alzheimer's disease. Radiat Res 2009;171:53–65.
105. Matanoski GM, Seltser R, Sartwell PE, et al. The current mortality rates of radiologists and other physician specialists: specific causes of death. Am J Epidemiol 1975;101:199–210.
106. Cardis E, Gilbert ES, Carpenter L, et al. Effects of low doses and low dose rates of external ionizing radiation: cancer mortality among nuclear industry workers in three countries. Radiat Res 1995;142:117–32.
107. Howe GR, Zablotska LB, Fix JJ, et al. Analysis of the mortality experience amongst U.S. nuclear power industry workers after chronic low-dose exposure to ionizing radiation. Radiat Res 2004;162:517–26.
108. Preston DL, Shimizu Y, Pierce DA, et al. Studies of mortality of atomic bomb survivors. Report 13: Solid cancer and noncancer disease mortality: 1950–1997. Radiat Res 2003;160:381–407.
109. Yamada M, Wong FL, Fujiwara S, et al. Noncancer disease incidence in atomic bomb survivors, 1958-1998. Radiat Res 2004;161:622–32.

110. US National Research Council, Committee to Assess Health Risks from Exposure to Low Level of Ionizing Radiation. Radiation-Induced Cancer: Mechanisms, Quantitative Experimental Studies, and the Role of Genetic Factors. Health risks from exposure to low levels of ionizing radiation: BEIR VII Phase 2. Washington (DC): National Academies Press; 2006. p. 65–90.
111. McDonald TA. A perspective on the potential health risks of PBDEs. Chemosphere 2002;46:745–55.
112. Imm P, Knobeloch L, Buelow C, et al. Household exposures to polybrominated diphenyl ethers (PBDEs) in a Wisconsin Cohort. Environ Health Perspect 2009;117: 1890–5.

The Aging Brain and Neurodegenerative Diseases

Gary W. Duncan, MD

KEYWORDS

- Aging • Neurodegenerative disease • Alzheimer's disease
- Parkinson's disease • Programmed cell death • Apoptosis
- Proteinopathies • Mitochondrial dysfunction
- Amyloid hypothesis • Biomarkers • Neuroimaging
- Risk factors for dementia

The successes of public and individual health accomplishments have lead to a greatly increased human lifespan. In the early 1900s, life expectancy was approximately 45 to 50 years; today individuals living into their 90s and even past 100 years are no longer considered unusual. This recent change of lifespan has therefore produced an increased number of older people. The greater the number of older people alive, the more people to experience changes associated with aging. Over the next decade, the number of older people will greatly increase, and thus the incidence of diseases associated with increased age will also increase. The incidence of neurodegenerative diseases common in older individuals has dramatically increased and has been predicted to increase even further as more and more baby boomers come in to their 60s and 70s. This article explores what is known about how the brain changes in normal aging and discuss more fully 2 important neurodegenerative diseases, Parkinson's disease (PD) and Alzheimer's disease (AD), seen in this aging brain setting.

The normal human life cycle includes changes in the body's function that progress as the age increases. Aging has been defined as the progressive loss of function accompanied by decreasing fertility and increasing mortality with advancing age.[1] This natural change associated with age is called senescence. Easily seen are the senescent changes in skin, hair, and body habitus. Similarly, senescence in nervous system organs and neurologic function also occurs. Several studies have documented actual changes in the neurologic examination that are not associated with disease and may be considered normal.[2–4] Examples of these findings include limited upgaze and downgaze, presbycusis, presbyopia, small and poorly reactive pupils,

Department of Neurology, Meharry Medical College, 1005 Dr D.B. Todd, Jr, Boulevard, Nashville, TN 37208, USA
E-mail address: gwduncan41@comcast.net

Clin Geriatr Med 27 (2011) 629–644
doi:10.1016/j.cger.2011.07.008
0749-0690/11/$ – see front matter © 2011 Elsevier Inc. All rights reserved.

geriatric.theclinics.com

slowed motor reaction time, muscle atrophy, reduction of tendon reflexes at the ankles, decreased sense of vibration, and changes in posture and gait.

This article examines more closely some of the senescent changes of the brain as well as common neurodegenerative changes. The latter are changes associated with diseases that increase in frequency with aging. These neurodegenerative diseases are characterized by progressive impairment of neuronal function and neuronal death in the brain; these processes are often localized in particular sites in the brain and thus the different diseases and syndromes produced by the neurodegenerative changes. In particular, brain changes in AD and PD and prevention attempts and strategies are discussed.

BRAIN CHANGES WITH AGING AND DISEASE

With age, the brain changes grossly and microscopically. Anatomic and magnetic resonance imaging studies have shown that with age the brain shrinks in size and there is increased size of the brain sulci and ventricles.[5,6] Contrary to previous thought, aging is not associated with marked neuronal loss; new methods of examining brain tissue have indicated that aging is more related to site-specific loss of complexity of the synaptic regions. The synapse region is a complex network of nerve terminals arrayed in 3 dimensions, allowing multiple sites of synaptic opportunities among many separate neurons. With aging, there is a reduction in terminal dendritic branching and in the density of the dendritic spines. This reduction in the complexity of the synapses reduces neuron to neuron communication.[7,8]

The mechanisms accounting for the changes in aging brains and diseased brains are receiving considerable research attention, particularly with the exploding advance in human survival. Aging of tissues, including the brain, and degenerative diseases are the result of progressive buildup of faulty cellular function and the resulting byproducts that are injurious to surrounding tissue. This process probably begins early in life. Also, earlier in life there are cellular mechanisms for repair of the faults and adequate responses to the stresses encountered. It is as if our cellular maintenance systems evolved to current state when our life expectancy was shorter, and our longer lifespans now out live the cellular defense mechanisms.[9] Several theories recently have been studied and postulated as causes of these phenomena. In general, the categories include external factors associated with aging, genetic factors, intracellular aging mechanisms, and programmed cell death (PCD). Certainly, one cannot entirely consider these categories as distinct; many explanations involve greater than or equal to 2 of them.

EXTERNAL FACTORS

How well an individual brain weathers the challenges of aging depends on many factors, including the environment, others diseases, exposures, and personal lifestyle. These random events that affect the brain may well test the genetic protection and general durability of the brain. External factors might hasten the cellular dysfunction and/or interfere with cellular maintenance and stress response mechanisms, thus increasing the adverse effects of aging or causing neurodegenerative diseases.

It is well known that nutrition is important for normal functioning of the body. Nutritional deficiencies such as B vitamins (B_1, B_3, and B_{12}) are known to cause symptomatic brain disease. Vitamin B_1 deficiency is associated with encephalopathy such as Wernicke's encephalopathy. Vitamin B_3 (niacin) deficiency causes dementia in the pellagra syndrome. Vitamin B_{12} has been postulated as a cause of dementia. However, none of these deficiencies are seen with any frequency in dementia in developed countries and are probably not part of normal aging or dementia. Stroke, infection, and head trauma can damage brain cells and can cause significant neurologic deficits that can lead to or cause a dementia picture. If they are involved in routine aging, it has not been proven yet. The effects of alcohol, smoking, and obesity are risk factors of disease that may affect the brain aging process, but the role any of these plays individually is not understood. Interestingly, smoking and use of caffeine have even been thought to be neuroprotective for PD.[10]

INTRACELLULAR AGING MECHANISMS
PCD

Brain cells can die owing to external injury or from internal mechanisms. External injuries typically cause necrosis of the cells. Injuries include hypoxia, trauma, and hypothermia.[11] With necrosis, the cells and intracellular organelles swell, the cell membrane breaks down, and cellular contents spill into the extracellular space.

Conversely, there are intracellular mechanisms that cause cells to die (PCD). The most common form of PCD is apoptosis. In contrast with necrosis, the histologic features of apoptosis include a morphologic change in which the neurons become round and shrink with membrane bleb formation, nuclear fragmentation, chromatin condensation, and loss of attachments. It represents a cell death in which the cell is an active participant; thus, it has been termed *cellular suicide*. Research has discovered many ways in which dysfunction of intracellular mechanisms lead to PCD. The dysfunctional mechanisms may occur in various parts of a neuron: Cell membrane, cytoplasm, mitochondria, nucleus, and endoplasmic reticulum. In several of the neurodegenerative diseases, the likely dysfunction site is known and understood to various degrees. Apoptosis can be initiated by external injury or stimuli such as heat, chemotherapeutic agents, or irradiation in dosages too low to cause outright necrosis.

Apoptosis plays a normal, vital role in many species, such as clearance of transitory cells in embryonic development, in normal cell turnover, and in tissue remodeling. Apoptosis also plays an important role in causation of neurodegenerative diseases when certain brain cells develop abnormal metabolism sufficient enough to prevent cell survival. Other forms of apoptosis include the following.

Proteinopathies

Many of the neurodegenerative diseases are caused by abnormal function or aggregation of intracellular proteins, which causes the particular brain cells to die; this process is called *proteinopathy*.[12] The protein aggregations may be in the cytoplasm as in PD, AD, or Huntington's disease, in the nucleus as in spinocerebellar ataxia type 1, in the endoplasmic reticulum as in as in a rare familial encephalopathy, or in the extracellular space as in AD. The aggregation of these proteins or the capacity of them to aggregate seems to be toxic to the neuron.

A small, 76-amino-acid protein (ubiquitin) is present in all eukaryotic cells, and is key in the degradation of intracellular proteins.[13] Ubiquitin is important in regulating protein metabolism by identifying specific proteins that need to be eliminated by enzymes called proteasomes. Malfunction of the ubiquitin system could prevent elimination of these irregular proteins, which could be toxic to neurons.

Another normal method of eliminating normal and abnormal proteins is *autophagy*.[13] Unneeded or unwanted proteins may be encapsulated in the cytoplasm and then auotphagocyzed and eliminated by the endoplasmic reticulum. This mechanism supplements the role of the proteasomes. Defects in this mechanism can lead to degenerative neuronal death and is involved in PCD.

Mitochondrial Dysfunction

Mitochondria are essential organelles for proper functioning of cells. Mitochondrial dysfunction can lead to degeneration and death of the cell. This mitochondrial dysfunction is thought to play a major role in the neurodegenerative diseases: AD, PD, Huntington's disease, and amyotrophic lateral sclerosis. Two types of mitochondrial function are thought to be important in neurodegenerative disease—mitochondrial DNA mutation and inability to adequately prevent accumulation of reactive oxygen species (ROS).[14] Mitochondrial-specific DNA can mutate and be less effective. There are known genetic diseases caused by inherited mutations in mitochondrial-specific DNA, including Kearns–Sayre syndrome, Leber hereditary optic neuropathy, and Pearson syndrome. With aging, there is an accumulation of mitochondrial-specific DNA that correlates with reduction of mitochondrial function.[14] The second type of dysfunction is a net increase of potentially harmful ROS. Mitochondria produce ROS as a byproduct of normal function, but they ordinarily also produce sufficient antioxidants to neutralize the ROS. With aging, mitochondrial damage results in an inability to neutralize the ROS resulting in net overproduction. This causes an increase in oxidative stress and damage to the brain, which has been implicated in causing aging related cognitive decline.[14,15]

Mitochondrial dysfunction and oxidative-induced damage play an important role in causation of AD, PD, Huntington's disease, and amyotrophic lateral sclerosis. These abnormal processes are related to the increased amount of β-amyloid in neurons and astrocytes, and they have been associated with activation of signaling patterns pathways that alter β-amyloid and τ-protein processing, and thus have a possible role in AD.[14] Mitochondrial dysfunction and oxidative stress also have been implicated in production of α-synuclein, which is the major component of Lewy bodies seen in PD.[14]

PARKINSON'S DISEASE

PD is a degenerative brain disease that occurs in the older population. PD has characteristic symptomatology and neuropathology. Although symptoms of the disease were described in ancient writings as early as 2000 to 4000 BC,[16] the constellation of symptoms was officially recognized in 1817 by James Parkinson.[17] Parkinson stressed the triad of akinesia, rigidity, and tremor as the symptoms and named the syndrome "shaking palsy." These 3 symptoms remain the characteristic triad of symptoms of PD. Subsequently, we have become aware of other symptoms of PD, some of which occur before the classic triad and some as the disease progresses.

The classic pathologic findings in PD include (1) loss of gross pigmentation in the substantia nigra and locus ceruleus, (2) loss of pigmented catecholaminergic neurons in the substantia nigra and locus ceruleus, (3) the presence of intracellular eosinophilic round inclusion bodies called Lewy bodies, and (4) cellular death in not only in these classically known areas but also of noradrenergic cells in the locus ceruleus, cholinergic cells in nucleus basalis of Meynert, and serotonergic cells in the raphe nucleus and autonomic nervous system.[18]

The pigmented cells of the substantia nigra and locus ceruleus manufacture dopamine, which is transported and released at synapses in the striatum (caudate nucleus, putamen, and globus pallidus in the basal ganglia). It is the lack of this neurotransmitter in the striatum that causes the characteristic symptoms. Fortunately, symptom modification can be effected with medicines. Orally administered dopamine cannot cross the blood–brain barrier, but when dopamine's precursor, L-dopa, is administered orally, it is absorbed by the gut, transported to brain by the circulation system, crosses the blood–brain barrier, and converted to dopamine in the striatum. Also, dopamine agonists can be administered and act at the postsynaptic sites in the striatum. Other commonly used drugs alter the amount of L-dopa that is delivered to the brain cells and the catabolism of dopamine in the brain. These agents are very successful at ameliorating symptoms, but do not significantly modify the disease process of PD. They do not cure the illness or alter progression of the disease process.

Symptoms of PD have been divided into those responsive to dopamine augmentation (dopaminergic) and those that are not responsive to dopamine augmentation (nondopaminergic). Dopaminergic symptoms include the classic triad symptoms of tremor, rigidity, and akinesia. Nondopaminergic symptoms include gait dysfunction with loss of postural balance, motor freezing, falling, autonomic nervous system disturbances, speech and swallowing disorders, sleep disturbance, mood alterations, and dementia.[19] Treatment of the dopaminergic symptoms has resulted in a major relief of symptoms and allowed prolonged active and useful life for patients with PD. However, in a long duration follow-up study, disability was more related to nondopaminergic symptoms, including falls (loss of central balance), autonomic disturbance, neuropsychiatric symptoms, and dementia.[20] There is no medicine to treat directly the nondopaminergic symptoms. Symptomatic treatment of the dementia, autonomic dysfunction, and neuropsychiatric symptoms is available.

The appearance of Lewy bodies in the brains of PD patients advances in a predictable sequence consisting of 5 stages.[18] It starts in the lower brain stem, autonomic nervous system, and olfactory bulb and nucleus in stages 1 and 2 and is associated with autonomic symptoms and loss of olfaction abilities. In stages 3 and 4, the Lewy bodies appear in substantia nigra and other nuclear areas of upper midbrain and forebrain; this is the during stage which motor symptoms occur. In stage 5, the Lewy bodies extend to the neocortex, and the complete picture of PD is present, including dementia. The loss of the cholinergic cells in the nucleus basalis of Meynert probably also contributes to dementia, and this explains why the cholinesterase inhibitors are successful at modifying the dementia symptoms of PD.

Currently, the clinical diagnosis of PD is established in stages 3 and 4 when characteristic dopaminergic motor symptoms occur. It is possible that nondopaminergic symptoms have a different time course and may appear earlier than the motor symptoms. There has been a recent attempt to identify the preclinical stages and premotor stages of PD. It is thought that neuronal dysfunction and death occurs begins approximately 5 years before onset of motor symptoms.[21] The preclinical stage would commence with the onset of neuronal dysfunction, and the premotor stage would begin with the death of the pigmented, dopaminergic cells in substantia nigra and locus ceruleus. In some of the small number of known genetic forms of PD, confirmation can be made by detection of abnormal genetic tests (the *parkin* gene). There is no blood test for idiopathic PD.

Neuroimaging currently offers the best method to screen and detect PD pathology in the brain. Neuroimaging studies designed to detect decreased dopamine in the substantia nigra have been successful in confirming the presence of PD. These imaging studies have demonstrated loss of [^{18}F]-flurodopa uptake in the contralateral putamen[22] and abnormal dopamine transporter SPECT scanning.[23] Because the scans would detect abnormal dopaminergic activity they could be useful in detecting the beginning of the premotor stage, that is, once the disease in the pigmented, dopaminergic cells has already begun. The scans would not be able to detect the nondopaminergic stage. These are the nondopaminergic symptoms mentioned plus

REM behavioral symptoms and decreased novelty seeking behavior.[24] Scanning relatives of patients with inherited PD has been successful in detecting which relatives will go on to develop PD.[25] Neuroimaging has also been able to detect characteristic PD abnormalities in normal people who have no family history of PD. However, too few studies are available to know whether neuroimaging will reliably detect asymptomatic patients who eventually will develop PD. The ability to recognize this "prodromal" stage would be of immense importance should safe, affordable, and effective neuroprotective agents for PD be developed. To detect persons susceptible to PD in these early stages with neuroimaging techniques would be monumental and very expensive. If disease modification were to be effective, there would have to be a practical, less expensive, and easily performed screening procedure. It is conceivable that screening for the nondopaminergic signs and symptoms might be a practical first step of early detection. For instance, detecting abnormal olfaction or diagnosing REM sleep behavior disorders might be part of a screening program.

Pathogenesis

Like all adult-onset neurodegenerative diseases, age is the major risk factor for PD. The cause of the progressive apoptosis of the pigmented neurons in the substantia nigra is not well understood. The hallmark Lewy body is composed primarily of the protein α-synuclein. As mentioned, proteins that are no longer needed or defective may be removed from the cell by the ubiquitin–proteasomes system and by autophagy. Abnormalities of these systems recently have been postulated to play a role in the formation of Lewy bodies from misfolded α-synuclein. The resulting buildup of α-synuclein leads to further aggregation of the protein to form the Lewy bodies, which seem to be toxic to neurons.[18] Mitochondrial dysfunction and oxidative stress have also been postulated as important in the apoptosis process.[26]

The pathologic etiology of PD is unclear. Most cases of PD have been considered non-hereditary (idiopathic); up to 15% are thought to be genetic. The idiopathic cases have long been thought to be related to some environmental factor(s). However, the knowledge that PD has been present for thousands of years and is present in various cultures and locations throughout the world make the causality of a single environmental toxin unlikely.[27] Head trauma and toxicity from MPTP (1-methyl-4-phenyl-1,2,3,6-tetrahydropyridine), manganese, and agricultural agents are thought to be causative external factors, but they represent a small number of cases of PD.

ALZHEIMER'S DISEASE

AD is a neurodegenerative disease that causes dementia. Dementia is a syndrome associated with progressive memory loss and greater than equal to 2 other cognitive impairments, such as language, orientation, judgment, planning, and calculation. Once dementia is diagnosed, evaluation must ensue to determine the etiology of the dementia. There are many causes of dementia; AD is the commonest cause of progressive dementia.

Dementia in its present understanding was first introduced in the 19th century by Philippe Pinel, a French physician, who has been described as the founder of modern psychiatry. Alois Alzheimer, in 1902, described the histologic findings in the brain of his patient, Augustine Deter, who had dementia. At autopsy Alzheimer examined the brain of Deter and identified amyloid plaques and neurofibrillary tangles (NFTs), which have become the histologic hallmarks of AD.

Amyloid plaques are amorphous deposits in the brain's interstitial space and consist of an insoluble form of β-amyloid protein (Aβ) with 40 and 42 amino acids in its center. There are inflammatory cells in the periphery of the plaques. The plaques' diameters are approximately 20 to 200 μm. These plaques are located in hippocampus, amygdala, and neocortex. The Aβ is derived from a protein called amyloid precursor protein (APP), a protein within the neuronal membrane that is involved in normal neuronal function. Ordinarily, APP is enzymatically cleaved by an α-secretase and a γ-secretase into a soluble Aβ, and this Aβ does not create plaques in the interstitial space. In AD, the APP is cleaved by β-secretase and later by γ-secretase, which produces insoluble Aβ that is the start of the amyloid plaque.[28] The Aβ deposits are thought to be toxic to the brain and thus may be the cause of AD (the amyloid hypothesis). The evidence for its causative role is multiple. First, the only early, genetic forms of AD have mutations of the APP and presenilins (secretases), which lead to the production of the insoluble Aβ42. Also, Aβ42 in the plaques has been demonstrated to be toxic to neurons in vitro. However, it may not be causative but a product of another, still unknown, etiology.

NFTs are intracellular filaments of hyperphosphorylated τ protein. One of the functions of τ protein is to stabilize neuronal intracellular microtubules, which transport materials from the neuronal cell body to the synaptic end of the neuron. In AD, the τ protein becomes hyperphosphorylated, and it is thought that this inhibits normal microtubule function.[29] This may be their role in the causation of AD.

Biomarkers

Many biomarkers that predict AD have been studied. These include brain atrophy as measured by magnetic resonance imaging software that measures brain volume, various chemicals in blood and cerebrospinal fluid (CSF), and detecting Aβ in the brain with neuroimaging. We discuss more fully 3 CSF markers and detection of brain Aβ with neuroimaging.

Measuring the amount of Aβ, total τ protein, and phosphorylated τ protein in CSF is becoming a valid test for the presence of AD. Recently, it has been shown that a combination of low CSF levels of Aβ1-42 and elevated levels of phosphorylated τ_{181P} has a diagnostic sensitivity of 90% for AD and a specificity of 64%. This combination of CSF biomarkers also can identify those with mild cognitive impairment (MCI) who will eventually develop AD. The same biomarkers were present in 39% of normal, nondemented subjects, which is a similar percentage of normal subjects who have amyloid plaques in their brains as detected by neuroimaging results and, also, by autopsy results. This finding suggests that these biomarkers may be useful in the diagnosis of AD in the presymptomatic stage. The same study also showed that the low Aβ is present in the asymptomatic subject and early in those with AD, and the level did not decrease further as the cognition progressively increased. On the other hand, the phosphorylated tau$_{181P}$ rose progressively along with progressive deterioration of cognition.

Recently, a neuroimaging technique that identifies brain Aβ protein aggregation in vivo has been introduced. The procedure uses positron emission tomography (PET) to detect ^{11}-carbon labeled Pittsburgh compound-B (PIB) attached to brain Aβ after intravenous injection.[30] The location in the brain of the detected signals corresponds with known brain sites of amyloid plaques in patients with AD, and it is presumed that this neuroimaging technique locates amyloid plaques in the brain. In clinically diagnosed AD patients, PET-PIB is positive in 80% to 100% of the cases. PET-PIB is positive in 10% to 30% of presumably normal controls, similar to the percentage of normal brains that have typical AD hallmarks at autopsy[31-34] and to the percentage of normal people having the CSF biomarkers mentioned.[35] Although it seems promising that PET-PIB in the future may be able to detect normal subjects likely to later develop AD, at this point the scans results must still be correlated with clinical evaluation. The PET-PIB is positive in 50% to 65% of patients with amnestic type MCI.[33,34] The few studies that have studied the relationship between positive PET-PPIB and conversion of MCI to AD show that PET-PIB has significant predictive value. Amyloid plaque buildup begins years before the onset of AD symptoms and probably reaches its maximum by the time symptoms are sufficient to make a clinical diagnosis.[35] Amyloid detection identifies those with AD and at risk for AD, but does not correlate with the degree of dementia. However, progression of dementia does correlate with ventricular expansion,[35] a sign of brain atrophy.

These biomarkers of AD are great scientific breakthroughs and will allow more accurate selection of patients with AD to study drugs and techniques to prevent and treat AD. The study groups will be purer by having patients with AD as defined by the biomarkers. Also, these biomarkers may provide a surrogate for determining the degree of prevention or effectiveness of treatments under consideration.

Treatment and Prevention

Currently, there are 5 agents for AD that have been approved by the US Food and Drug Administration. Four are acetylcholine esterase inhibitors—tacrine, donepezil, rivastigmine, and razadyne—and 1 an N-methyl-D-aspartic acid (NMDA) blocker (mementine). These agents are all designed for symptom modification and do not modify the disease.

There is an imperative to seek a strategy for prevention and/or treatment of dementia because of the alarming increasing incidence and prevalence of the disease and because of the devastating effects of the disease on individuals and their families. Assuming the amyloid cascade is the correct etiology for AD, then an agent that interferes with production of amyloid deposition or one that hastens its removal from the brain would be the best treatment as well as the best preventative for those who are found to have asymptomatic amyloid deposition. We currently do not have such agents available.

Presuming that the deposition of an abundance of insoluble Aβ is crucial in the etiology of AD, any disease modification attempt for prevention or treatment must include strategies to either prevent the Aβ from aggregating in the amyloid plaques or removing the Aβ after amyloid plaques have already been formed. Lifestyle modifications or medicines that could accomplish either of these objective might be able to prevent AD or modify the disease if already established.

Prevention of Amyloid Plaque Formation

As mentioned, abnormal cleavage of the transmembrane APP by β- and γ-secretases produces the insoluble Aβ that leads to amyloid plaque formation. β-Secretase is widespread, and safe inhibitors have not been brought to clinical trials. γ-Secretase modulators change the action of the secretase so that insoluble Aβ is not formed. At the time of writing, a γ-secretase modulator (tarenflurbil,[36] a nonsteroidal anti-inflammatory agent) and a γ-secretase inhibitor (semagacestat; unpublished data) have been compared with placebo in large, phase III randomized controlled trials (RCTs) and have not been shown to be beneficial. The studies were halted after preliminary data review. Another approach at preventing plaque formation is to prevent the Aβ from forming amyloid plaques, even if it has been produced by abnormal cleavage of APP. One anti-aggregating agent, tramiprosate, has also been tried in a phase III study without demonstrated efficacy, and the study was terminated. Other γ-secretases and anti-aggregating agents currently are under study.

Removing Aβ From Brain

In mice genetically engineered to progressively develop amyloid plaques early in life, active immunization with Aβ has successfully prevented the new formation of amyloid plaques and removed those already present at the time of immunization.[37] Active immunization in these types of experimental animals also seemed to attenuate the behavioral changes associated with the amyloid plaque formation.[38,39] These results gave hope that active immunization of AD patients might rid the brains of plaque and cause improvement in cognitive skills. However, the first clinical trial with active immunization with full-length Aβ was accompanied with serious meningoencephalitis, and the study had to be terminated.[40] Second-generation, active vaccines with better safety profiles have been developed and are being tested. In addition, passive immunization by directly infusing antibodies against Aβ is being researched.[41]

The thought that the formation and deposition of the amyloid protein is the most likely cause of AD has been the focus of much of the research on etiology and treatment of AD. Many scientists are devoting a lot of time and money to finding a way to prevent amyloid production. As mentioned, at least 4 drugs designed to interfere with the amyloid hypothesis thus far have not been successful in RCTs. Some investigators have maintained that the amyloid plaques are not the cause of AD, but are the consequence of AD development, or that in some way the formation of amyloid plaques may be part of a protective strategy of the brain. The amyloid hypothesis may be losing some of its underpinnings as the cause of AD and the target of drugs and agents to prevent and treat AD, but much research is still continuing.

Preventing NFT Formation

Less research on interfering with formation of NFT has been published.

RISK FACTORS AND PREVENTION OF DEMENTIA

Understanding the complexity of the normal changes in the aging brain and those we know about in neurodegenerative disease, one can understand the difficulty to develop lifestyle changes or other medications that would prevent or alter the progression of AD and other dementias. We have knowledge of increased ROS accumulation associated with mitochondrial dysfunction, abnormal APP and secretase activity in cell membranes, deposition of amyloid protein in brain, and inflammatory cells in the amyloid plaques. In addition, we know that vascular risk factors (VRFs) play a role in vascular dementia and probably also in AD; at least, they seem to increase severity of dementia and timing of onset of symptoms.[42] This knowledge gives credence to attempts to develop diets, medicines, vitamin supplementations, and physical, cognitive, and social activities that might prevent or slow down the aging and neurodegenerative changes. Theoretically, AD is an ideal disease to prevent, because there is such a prolonged period of asymptomatic time in the individual's earlier years during which there are no pathologic AD changes in the brain. Treatment of the disease once symptoms are present might not be successful; ideally, patients could be identified in the asymptomatic phase and treated at a time when the treatment might be successful.[43]

Genetic risk factors for late onset AD include the presence of 2 alleles of E4 variety of the apolipoprotein E (ApoE) gene and trisomy 21 (Down syndrome). ApoE is a normal lipoprotein in the body. There are several forms of ApoE (ApoE2, ApoE3, and ApoE4) When both of the gene's alleles are the E4 variety, there is an increased risk of atherosclerosis and of AD. Finding the double E4 only recognizes a group of individuals with a higher than normal risk for AD and does not indicate that an

vitamin C, folate, beta carotene, or a diet low in saturated fat and high in vegetable intake. So far, RCTs have not documented any value of vitamin supplementation, gingko biloba co-administered with vitamin E, or ω-3 fatty acids supplementation in preventing cognitive decline. Smoking, but not past history of smoking, is associated with increased risk for cognitive decline.

They noted consistent association of cognitive decline with hypertension and modest correlation with diabetes and the metabolic syndrome. However, most trials of antihypertensive treatment did not result in cognitive benefit. Likewise, they did not find any evidence for giving estrogen, gonadal steroids, or cholinesterase inhibitors. There was a lack of high-quality studies looking at the effect of sleep apnea, traumatic brain injury, and obesity. Depression and depressive symptoms have been associated with MCI and cognitive decline. No consistent evidence is present for an association with drugs such as statins, antihypertensive medications or anti-inflammatory drugs.

Early life socioeconomic status, cognitive milieu, years of education, living alone, or being without a partner have limited or no consistent association with cognitive decline. However, they noted that the loss of a spouse was robustly associated with cognitive decline. They point out that increase involvement in cognitive activity may be related to slower decline in cognition and lower risk for cognitive impairment. A large randomized trial of cognitive training over 5 to 6 weeks with booster training later, has shown a small, significant reduction of cognitive decline over a 5-year period. There is little evidence that increased physical therapy or aerobic activity improves or maintains cognition. Likewise, they did not find any evidence for giving estrogen, gonadal steroids, or cholinesterase inhibitors.

SUMMARY

The effects of aging on the brain are numerous and are just beginning to be understood; much remains to be discovered. After a glacial-like pace of development of our knowledge of the effects of aging on the brain and the production of neurodegenerative disease in the last century, research now is providing us with new knowledge at a rapid pace. Almost daily or weekly, new important contributions to our knowledge appear. The current burden to individuals, families, and to our economy is large, but the potential burden with the aging of the world's population likely will be monumental.

The neurodegenerative diseases remain a therapeutic enigma despite the explosion of new and exciting scientific knowledge about them. We understand the chemical content and to some degree the development of the previously poorly understood histologic hallmarks of PD and AD, but still we do not firmly understand the relationship between these proteinaceous brain deposits and the causation of the diseases. The theory that development and deposition of amyloid protein in the brain (amyloid hypothesis) causes AD has been the focus for most of the research of etiology and treatment of the disease. The recent failure of several large RCTs investigating drugs that modify the formation of amyloid plaques has shaken the underpinnings of the amyloid hypothesis, but certainly has not negated it or prevented further investigation of therapeutic approaches based on the theory. Regrettably, even though we have knowledge of some AD risk factors, research into the therapeutic value of treating risk factors or of manipulating lifestyles to prevent or modify neurodegenerative disease is difficult and has not been conclusive.

We are near to the point that we can diagnose presymptomatic PD and AD, and we eagerly await effective treatments and prevention strategies for them and other neurodegenerative diseases. The recognized risk factors for AD are also risk factors for cardiovascular and cerebrovascular disease, and the effectiveness of treating them in preventing these conditions is established. For now, the primary care physician should redouble efforts to detect and treat these risk factors, not only for their proven value to the health of patients, but also for the possibility that the effort is important in preventing neurodegenerative diseases.

REFERENCES

1. Kirkwood TBL, Austad SN. Why do we age? Nature 2000;408:233–8.
2. Ropper A, Samuels M. The Neurology of Aging. New York: The McGraw-Hill; 2005.
3. Jenkyn LR, Reeves AG, Warren T, et al. Neurologic signs in senescence. Arch Neurol 1985;42:1154–7.
4. Benassi G, D'Alessandro R, Gallassi R, et al. Neurological examination in subjects over 65 years: an epidemiological survey. Neuroepidemiology 1990;9:27–38.
5. Esiri M, Hyman B, Beyreuther K, et al, editors. Ageing and Dementia. 6th edition. London: Arnold; 1997.
6. DeCarli C, Massaro J, Harvey D, et al. Measures of brain morphology and infarction in the Framingham Heart Study: establishing what is normal. Neurobiol Aging 1997;26: 491–510.
7. Burke SN, Barnes CA. Neural plasticity in the ageing brain. Nat Rev Neurosci 2006;7:30–40.
8. Lister JP, Barnes CA. Neurobiological changes in the hippocampus during normative aging. Arch Neurol 2009 2009;66:829–33.
9. Kirkwood TBL. The most pressing problem of our age. BMJ 2003;326:1297–9.
10. Bernedetti MD, Bower JH, Maraganore D. Smoking, alcohol and coffee consumption preceding Parkinson's disease. Neurology 2000;55:1350–8.
11. Bredesen D, Rammohan V, Mehlen P. Cell death in the nervous system. Nature 2006;443:796–802.
12. Taylor J, Fischbeck K. Toxic proteins in neurodegenerative disease. Science 2002; 296:1991–5.
13. Rubinsztein D. The roles of intracellular protein-degradation pathways in neurodegeneration. Nature 2006;443:780–6.
14. Lin M, Beal M. Mitochondrial dysfunction and oxidative stress in neurodegenerative diseases. Nature 2006;443:787–95.
15. Lu T, Pan Y, Kao S, et al. Gene regulation and DNA damage in the ageing human brain. Nature 2004;429:883–91.
16. Westerlund M, Hoffer B, Olson L. Parkinson's disease: exit toxins, enter genetics. Prog Neurobiol 2010;90:146–56.
17. Parkinson J. An essay on the shaking palsy. London: Sherwood; 1817.
18. Braak H, Ghebremedhin E, Rub U, et al. Stages in the development of Parkinson's disease-related pathology. Cell Tissue Res 2004;318:121–34.
19. Olanow C, Kieburtz K, Schapira A. Why have we failed to achieve neuroprotection in Parkinson's disease? Ann Neurol 2008;64:S101–10.
20. Hely M, Morris J, Reid W, et al. Sydney Multicenter Study of Parkinson's disease: non-L-dopa-responsive problems. Mov Disord 2005;20:190–9.
21. Fearnley J, Lees A. Ageing and Parkinson's disease: substantia nigra regional selectivity. Brain 1991;114:2283–301.
22. Morrish P, Sawle G, Brooks D. Clinical and [18F] dopa PET findings in early Parkinson's disease. J Neurol Neurosurg Psychiatry 1995;59:597–600.
23. Marek K, Seibyl J, Zoghbi S, et al. [123I] beta-CIT/SPECT imaging demonstrates bilateral loss of dopamine. Neurology 1996;46:231–7.

24. Menza MA, Mark MH, Burn DJ, et al. Personality correlates of [18F]dopa striatal uptake: results of positron-emission tomography in Parkinson's disease. J Neuropsychiatry Clin Neurosci 1995;7:176–9.

25. Piccini P, Burn DJ, Ceravolo R, et al. The role of inheritance in sporadic Parkinson's disease: evidence from a longitudinal study of dopaminergic function in twins. Ann Neurol 1999;45:577–82.

26. Spillantini M, Crowther R, Jakes R, et al. alpha-Synuclein in filamentous inclusions of Lewy bodies from Parkinson's disease. Proc Natl Acad Sci U S A 1998;95:6469–73.

27. Abou-Sleiman P, Muqit M, Wood N. Expanding insights of mitochondrial dysfunction in Parkinson's disease. Nat Rev Neurosci 2006;7:207–19.

28. Hardy J, Allsop D. Amyloid deposition as the central event in the aetiology of Alzheimer's disease. Trends Pharmacol Sci 1991;12:383–8.

29. Cowan CM, Chee F, Shepherd D, et al. Disruption of neuronal function by soluble hyperphosphorylated tau in a Drosophila model of tauopathy. Biochem Soc Trans 2010;38:564–70.

30. Klunk WE, Engler H, Nordberg A, et al. Imaging brain amyloid in Alzheimer's disease with Pittsburgh compound-B. Ann Neurol 2004;55:306–19.

31. Rowe CC, Ng S, Ackermann U, et al. Imaging beta-amyloid burden in aging and dementia. Neurology 2007;68:1718–25.

32. Edison P, Archer HA, Hinz R, et al. Amyloid, hypometabolism, and cognition in Alzheimer disease: an [11C]PIB and [18F]FDG PET study. Neurology 2007;68:501–8.

33. Wolk DA, Klunk W. Update on amyloid imaging: from healthy aging to Alzheimer's disease. Curr Neurol Neurosci Rep 2009;9:345–52.

34. Wolk DA, Price JC, Saxton JA, et al. Amyloid imaging in mild cognitive impairment subtypes. Ann Neurol 2009;65:557–68.

35. Jack CR Jr, Lowe VJ, Weigand SD, et al. Serial PIB and MRI in normal, mild cognitive impairment and Alzheimer's disease: implications for sequence of pathological events in Alzheimer's disease. Brain 2009;132:1355–65.

36. Green RC, Schneider LS, Amato DA, et al. Effect of tarenflurbil on cognitive decline and activities of daily living in patients with mild Alzheimer disease: a randomized controlled trial. JAMA 2009;302:2557–64.

37. Schenk D, Barbour R, Dunn W, et al. Immunization with amyloid-beta attenuates Alzheimer-disease-like pathology in the PDAPP mouse. Nature 1999;400:173–7.

38. Janus C, Pearson J, McLaurin J, et al. A beta peptide immunization reduces behavioural impairment and plaques in a model of Alzheimer's disease. Nature 2000;408:979–82.

39. Morgan D, Diamond DM, Gottschall PE, et al. A beta peptide vaccination prevents memory loss in an animal model of Alzheimer's disease. Nature 2000;408:982–5.

40. Gilman S, Koller M, Black RS, et al. Clinical effects of Abeta immunization (AN1792) in patients with AD in an interrupted trial. Neurology 2005;64:1553–62.

41. Town T. Alternative Abeta immunotherapy approaches for Alzheimer's disease. CNS Neurol Disord Drug Targets 2009;8:114–27.

42. Snowdon DA, Greiner LH, Mortimer JA, et al. Brain infarction and the clinical expression of Alzheimer disease. The Nun Study. JAMA 1997;277:813–7.

43. Mohajeri MH, Leuba G. Prevention of age-associated dementia. Brain Res Bull 2009;80:315–25.

44. Middleton LE, Yaffe K. Promising strategies for the prevention of dementia. Arch Neurol 2009;66:1210–5.

45. Fillit H, Nash DT, Rundek T, et al. Cardiovascular risk factors and dementia. Am J Geriatr Pharmacother 2008;6:100–18.

46. Ott A, Stolk RP, van Harskamp F, et al. Diabetes mellitus and the risk of dementia: The Rotterdam Study. Neurology 1999;53:1937.

47. Yaffe K, Blackwell T, Kanaya AM, et al. Diabetes, impaired fasting glucose, and development of cognitive impairment in older women. Neurology 2004;63:658–63.

48. Luchsinger JA. Adiposity, hyperinsulinemia, diabetes and Alzheimer's disease: an epidemiological perspective. Eur J Pharmacol 2008;585:119–29.

49. Yaffe K. Metabolic syndrome and cognitive disorders: is the sum greater than its parts? Alzheimer Dis Assoc Disord 2007;21:167–71.

50. Launer LJ, Masaki K, Petrovitch H, et al. The association between midlife blood pressure levels and late-life cognitive function: The Honolulu-Asia Aging Study. JAMA 1995;274:1846–51.

51. Qiu C, Winblad B, Fratiglioni L. The age-dependent relation of blood pressure to cognitive function and dementia. Lancet Neurol 2005;4:487–99.

52. Prince MJ, Bird AS, Blizard RA, et al. Is the cognitive function of older patients affected by antihypertensive treatment? Results from 54 months of the Medical Research Council's trial of hypertension in older adults. BMJ 1996;312:801–5.

53. Muldoon MF, Ryan CM, Sereika SM, et al. Randomized trial of the effects of simvastatin on cognitive functioning in hypercholesterolemic adults. Am J Med 2004;117:823–9.

54. Morris MC, Evans DA, Tangney CC, et al. Associations of vegetable and fruit consumption with age-related cognitive change. Neurology 2006;67:1370–6.

55. Engelhart MJ, Geerlings MI, Ruitenberg A, et al. Dietary intake of antioxidants and risk of Alzheimer disease. JAMA 2002;287:3223–9.

56. Barberger-Gateau P, Raffaitin C, Letenneur L, et al. Dietary patterns and risk of dementia: the Three-City cohort study. Neurology 2007;69:1921–30.

57. Kang JH, Ascherio A, Grodstein F. Fruit and vegetable consumption and cognitive decline in aging women. Ann Neurol 2005;57:713–20.

58. Morris MC, Evans DA, Bienias JL, et al. Consumption of fish and n-3 fatty acids and risk of incident Alzheimer disease. Arch Neurol 2003 2003;60:940–6.

59. Morris MC, Beckett LA, Scherr PA, et al. Vitamin E and vitamin C supplement use and risk of incident Alzheimer disease. Alzheimer Dis Assoc Disord 1998;12:121–6.

60. Masaki KH, Losonczy KG, Izmirlian G, et al. Association of vitamin E and C supplement use with cognitive function and dementia in elderly men. Neurology 2000;54:1265–72.

61. Commenges D, Scotet V, Renaud S, et al. Intake of flavonoids and risk of dementia. Eur J Epidemiol 2000;16:357–63.

62. Morris MC, Evans DA, Bienias JL, et al. Dietary intake of antioxidant nutrients and the risk of incident Alzheimer disease in a biracial community study. JAMA 2002;287:3230–7.

63. Foley DJ, White LR. Dietary intake of antioxidants and risk of Alzheimer disease: food for thought. JAMA 2002;287:3261–3.

64. Luchsinger JA, Tang MX, Shea S, et al. Antioxidant vitamin intake and risk of Alzheimer disease. Arch Neurol 2003;60:203–8.

65. Zandi PP, Anthony JC, Khachaturian AS, et al. Reduced risk of Alzheimer disease in users of antioxidant vitamin supplements: the Cache County Study. Arch Neurol 2004;61:82–8.

66. Dunn JE, Weintraub S, Stoddard AM, et al. Serum alpha-tocopherol, concurrent and past vitamin E intake, and mild cognitive impairment. Neurology 2007;68:670–6.

67. Yaffe K, Clemons TE, McBee WL, et al. Impact of antioxidants, zinc, and copper on cognition in the elderly: a randomized, controlled trial. Neurology 2004;63:1705–7.

68. Petersen RC, Thomas RG, Grundman M, et al. Vitamin E and donepezil for the treatment of mild cognitive impairment. N Engl J Med 2005;352:2379–88.

69. Kang JH, Cook N, Manson J, et al. A randomized trial of vitamin E supplementation and cognitive function in women. Arch Intern Med 2006;166:2462–8.

70. Kang JH, Cook NR, Manson JE, et al. Vitamin E, vitamin C, beta carotene, and cognitive function among women with or at risk of cardiovascular disease: The Women's Antioxidant and Cardiovascular Study. Circulation 2009;119:2772–80.

71. Gu Y, Nieves JW, Stern Y, et al. Food combination and Alzheimer disease risk: a protective diet. Arch Neurol 2010;67:699–706.

72. Rolland Y, Abellan van Kan G, et al. Physical activity and Alzheimer's disease: from prevention to therapeutic perspectives. J Am Med Dir Assoc 2008;9:390–405.

73. Rockwood K, Middleton L. Physical activity and the maintenance of cognitive function. Alzheimers Dement 2007;3(2 Suppl):S38–44.

74. Stern Y. Cognitive reserve and Alzheimer disease. Alzheimer Dis Assoc Disord 2006;20(3 Suppl 2):S69–74.

75. Carlson MC, Helms MJ, Steffens DC, et al. Midlife activity predicts risk of dementia in older male twin pairs. Alzheimers Dement 2008;4:324–31.

76. Fratiglioni L, Wang HX. Brain reserve hypothesis in dementia. J Alzheimers Dis 2007;12:11–22.

77. Acevedo A, Loewenstein DA. Nonpharmacological cognitive interventions in aging and dementia. J Geriatr Psychiatry Neurol 2007;20:239–49.

78. Ball K, Berch DB, Helmers KF, et al. Effects of cognitive training interventions with older adults: a randomized controlled trial. JAMA 2002;288:2271–81.

79. Neugroschl J, Sano M. Current treatment and recent clinical research in Alzheimer's disease. Mt Sinai J Med 2010;77:3–16.

80. Henderson VW, Paganini-Hill A, Miller BL, et al. Estrogen for Alzheimer's disease in women: randomized, double-blind, placebo-controlled trial. Neurology 2000;54:295–301.

81. Mulnard RA, Cotman CW, Kawas C, et al. Estrogen replacement therapy for treatment of mild to moderate Alzheimer disease: a randomized controlled trial. Alzheimer's Disease Cooperative Study. JAMA 2000;283:1007–15.

82. Craig MC, Maki PM, Murphy DG. The Women's Health Initiative Memory Study: findings and implications for treatment. Lancet Neurol 2005;4:190–4.

83. Maki PM, Gast MJ, Vieweg AJ, et al. Hormone therapy in menopausal women with cognitive complaints: a randomized, double-blind trial. Neurology 2007;69:1322–30.

84. Daviglus ML, Bell CC, Berrettini W, et al. National Institutes of Health State-of-the-Science Conference Statement: preventing alzheimer disease and cognitive decline. Ann Intern Med 2010;153:176–81.

Psychosocial Factors in Aging

Michele M. Larzelere, PhD[a],*,
James Campbell, MD[a], Nana Yaw Adu-Sarkodie, MD, MPH[b]

KEYWORDS

• Psychology • Aging • Personality • Religiosity
• Social relationships • Ageism

PSYCHOSOCIAL FACTORS IN AGING

How old would you be if you didn't know how old you were?

—Satchel Paige

Aging is often portrayed as a decline into physical limitation and psychological misery. Although aging presents challenges, advances in biopsychosocial care are extending the active and vital portion of the lifespan. Individual physical, social, and psychological factors impact the rate at which "old age" is "felt," leaving age alone as a largely nonspecific indicator of a person's physical, cognitive, and psychological status. On the one hand, for individuals who age with good health, the "young" old period, which is defined from the late-50s to mid-70s is, in large part, an extension of psychological middle age. Frailty/poor health in this age group is, on the other hand, associated with significant declines in psychological well-being.[1]

The United States Census Bureau projects that there will be 88 million Americans older than the age of 65 years by 2050, of whom 19 million will be older than age 85.[2] It is likely that fewer than 50% of the "oldest old" (>85) will lack significant disability.[3] In addition, it is estimated that by 2050, 36% of elders in the United States will be non-Caucasian (both native born and immigrants).[2] This statistic has significant implications for understanding and predicting the impact of aging, as members of minority groups are often burdened with poorer health at younger ages.[4] It is important to note that low socioeconomic status and level of education have both been associated with increased mortality among the elderly.[5] Education also plays a significant role.[6] For example, it is estimated that college education can delay the

The authors have nothing to disclose.
[a] Family Medicine Residency, Louisiana State University Health Sciences Center, 200 West Esplanade Avenue, Kenner, LA 70065, USA
[b] Louisiana State University Health Sciences Center Geriatrics Fellowship, 200 West Esplanade Avenue, Kenner, LA 70065, USA
* Corresponding author.
E-mail address: mlarze@lsuhsc.edu

impact of aging by nearly one decade (eg, college-educated individuals reached equivalent levels of death and disability approximately one decade after those with less education).[7]

Although disparities in illness burden cause minorities and those of lower socio-economic status to become impaired at younger ages,[8] health decline does not always indicate poor life quality. For both genders and all races, happy life years exceed disability-free life years,[9] and a majority of seniors (>75%) consider themselves to be aging very successfully (even though they might not meet objective standards for optimal aging).[10] Although demographic factors such as minority status, immigrant status, and socioeconomic and educational achievement cannot be altered to help seniors age more successfully, many psychosocial factors can be impacted. This article explores some of the factors associated with positive biopsychosocial aging.

ATTITUDES ABOUT AGING

In 1981, Silverstein wrote, "The Little Boy and the Old Man":

Said the little boy, "Sometimes I drop my spoon."

Said the little old man, "I do that too."

The little boy whispered, "I wet my pants."

"I do that too," laughed the little old man.

Said the little boy, "I often cry."

The old man nodded, "So do I."

"But worst of all," said the boy, "it seems

Grown-ups don't pay attention to me."

And he felt the warmth of the wrinkled old hand.

"I know what you mean," said the little old man.[11]

This poem depicts the way in which society marginalizes its most senior and most junior members. Adults of all ages generally believe that good traits are lost through aging, unwelcome changes occur, and decline is uncontrollable.[12] Six common aging myths debunked by Rowe and Kahn (1998)[3] are summarized in **Table 1**.

The types of stereotypical attitudes listed in **Table 1** can lead to undue emotional stress among the elderly and to self-defeating behaviors.[17] The impact of aging stereotypes on seniors' self-perceptions has been explained through the use of labeling theory. According to labeling theory, ageism would lead a younger person to perceive older adults as less capable or negative in some other manner. This causes negative self-perceptions in older adults and a concomitant decline in self-esteem. For example, a young caregiver may berate his or her older charge. The older adult may, in turn, adopt the negative views and act accordingly, with detrimental effects to his or her self-image and functioning.[18]

Research has largely supported labeling theory. For example, it has been shown that stereotypes tend to diminish a person's basic sense of worth. Levy[19] found that those exposed to negative stereotypes exhibited reduced memory performance, decreased self-efficacy, and a decline in will to live. Fortunately, it has been demonstrated that simple awareness that a stereotype has been activated can

Table 1
Aging myths and realities[11]

Myth	Reality
1. To be old is to be sick.	The majority of older adults are able to perform functions necessary for daily living and to manage independently until they are in very advanced ages, despite increasing chronic illness and disability.[3]
2. You can't teach an old dog new tricks.	As it relates to cognitive vitality and the adoption of new behaviors, older people are indeed capable of learning new things. Many older adults who live into their 90s retain high cognitive function, and several population-based studies have suggested that 15%–30% of centenarians remain cognitively intact.[13]
3. The horse is out of the barn.	It is never too late to gain benefits from health-promoting behaviors, such as increasing physical activity.[11] This has implications for how health providers approach preventive health messages for the elderly.
4. The secret to successful aging is to choose your parents wisely.	Social and behavioral factors play a larger role in one's overall health status and functioning than genetic factors. Health and well-being are affected by preventive behaviors, including cancer screenings and vaccinations, as well as by diet, physical activity, obesity, cigarette smoking, social interactions and attachments, and the air quality where people live.[14]
5. The lights are on, but the voltage is low.	The majority of older people with partners and without major health problems are sexually active. According to Dunn,[15] older adults find sexual activity to be pleasurable and life affirming; the need for physical closeness and intimacy does not diminish with age. If intercourse is no longer possible due to physical ailments, caressing, stroking, and kissing are often emotionally gratifying activities that can give sensual pleasure and will be accepted if the physician presents them as normal variations in sexual activity.[15]
6. The elderly don't pull their own weight.	The majority of older adults who do not earn wages are engaged in some form of productive role within their families or the community at large. Many seniors care for younger family members and participate in volunteer activities. Further, in 2002, 30% of individuals who remained economically active after age 70 held professional and managerial jobs, presumably using the skills and knowledge developed during long careers. Another 17% worked in the service sector, with somewhat smaller percentages engaged as craftsmen/operatives and as manual laborers.[16]

suppress stereotype-consistent behavior, providing us with a remedy for the ageism that is pervasive in society.[20]

To maintain positive self-perceptions, older adults must overcome the effects of organic change and the barrage of negative ageist stereotypes. Goldman and Goldman (1981)[21] suggest that as people grow older, their attitudes toward old age become more negative. Other authors[22] have found that the attitudes of elderly people toward their own age group are more positive than the attitudes of the young toward them. Ron[23] suggests that the attitudes of people are formulated at an early age and that life experiences and family–cultural perceptions have an effect on these perceptions. Kaufman relates that elderly people experience the self as disconnected from age and that those who held positive or negative attitudes toward old age and aging in the past will not likely change their mind (today) in their old age.[24] Plainly, biases about older people become aging self-stereotypes in old age, and preventive intervention for age stereotyping is to form realistic aging stereotypes well before one becomes old.[25]

Elders' aging self-perceptions have the capacity to affect a variety of health outcomes beneficially, including functional health over time, survival, and will to live.[26] In a retrospective analysis of data captured by the Ohio Longitudinal Study of Aging and Retirement, Levy and Myers found that individuals who had more positive self-perceptions of aging were significantly more likely to practice preventive health behaviors, and that aging self-perceptions had a greater impact on health behaviors than any of the other covariate controls, including alcohol consumption, diet, exercise, medication compliance, seatbelt use, tobacco use, as well as regular physician visits.[27] Seniors with negative self-perceptions may benefit from interventions designed to make their judgments more healthy and adaptive.[28]

Professionals also need to confront their own biases and stereotypes about aging to serve elders effectively. Medical ageism, in particular, is important because it can lead to a tendency to give less aggressive treatments based on age characteristics alone.[29] For example, medical ailments in the elderly are often not taken as seriously or are at times even misdiagnosed and attributed to old age.[30] Greene and colleagues (1989) showed that physicians provided less-detailed medical information to older patients.[29] Physicians who are uncomfortable with their own aging or who lack knowledge of special geriatric issues often miss opportunities to diagnose and offer appropriate therapies for geriatric conditions.[31] Some interventions that may be useful include individuating elders (emphasizing each senior's individual personality traits and abilities), and increasing younger medical providers' exposure to older adults, which leads to improved knowledge about aging and decreased belief in negative stereotypes about aging.[32]

SOCIAL RELATIONSHIPS

Grow old with me! The best is yet to be.

—Robert Browning

One of the most popular lenses through which social relationships of seniors are viewed is the socioemotional selectivity theory (SST). The SST postulates that the nature of social interactions and relationships changes over time.[33] As the perception of time remaining in life becomes more limited, individuals become more focused on emotional satisfaction in their social interactions, and focus less on gaining knowledge and information. As people progress through life, they devote more attention to their present situation, and concentrate less on future development, resulting in actions that tend to promote their own emotional stability. Through facilitation of favorable emotional experiences, the elderly attempt to construct social networks that minimize adverse emotional interaction. Thus, in old age, peripheral interpersonal relationships are selectively decreased, and established, familiar, meaningful relationships and social activities, as with family and old friends, grow in importance and emphasis.

Several studies have demonstrated a greater proportion of positive memories to mixed stimuli among older adults, which is congruent with socioemotional selectivity theory (SST).[34] One randomized controlled trial (RCT) found more efficient mood repair (restoration of positive mood) in older adults, supporting SST.[35] Another RCT demonstrated enhanced recollection of emotional memories following emotional cues in older adults, again, supportive of SST.[36] A 2009 study of self-reported social attachment tendencies in 200 subjects showed a lower frequency of troubled relationships in older versus younger participants, lending some credence to the SST hypothesis of improved relationships in older adults over time.[37] Older adults have also been shown to decrease their involvement in organizations that are less important to them and to maintain a high level of volunteerism with the organizations they find most meaningful, which supports SST precepts.[38]

In the face of such positive evidence, a number of published studies contradict the principles of SST.[39] These studies suggest that it is the presence of limited time, not aging per se, that produces the results predicted by SST.

Social Support

There is sound epidemiological and demographic evidence to support a positive correlation between social integration and positive health benefits.[40] The 5-year mortality rate in men with no social ties is 160 per 1000, compared to 70 per 1000 in men with two social ties. Similar data in women indicate rates of 70 per 1000 with no social ties, and 45 per 1000 with two social ties. Statistics reflect additional reductions in mortality with increasing numbers of social ties.[34] Socially integrated people have lower incidence of physical illnesses, both serious (cancer recurrence[41]) and minor (upper respiratory infections[42]). Decreased stroke incidence,[43] less arterial calcification,[44] and lower overall mortality[45] have also been demonstrated among socially integrated individuals with cardiovascular disease (or cardiovascular risk), compared to those individuals with fewer social ties.

The existence of an established social support system reduces morbidity due not only to physical illness, but mental illnesses as well.[46] Individuals with strong social support networks report greater resiliency to stressors and improved general emotional well-being.[47] Seniors who perceive strong social support in their lives are at decreased risk for suicidal ideation.[48] However, social connections are not universally positive. There can also be situational adverse physical and mental health effects associated with social relationships, largely dependent on the quality and demands of those relationships.[20,49] Dysfunctional or nonsupportive relationships have been linked to higher rates of depression and decreased sense of well-being in the older population.[50]

Several studies have demonstrated improved health status through interventions that facilitate social interaction. An RCT published in 1995 showed that veterans enrolled in a geriatric evaluation and management program reported higher rates of social interaction compared to a control group, and mortality rates in the treatment group were 54% lower.[51] Another RCT studied 235 adults older than age 74, and demonstrated improved survival through a social integration program at day care centers.[52] A 2002 longitudinal Swedish population-based study showed decreased risk of dementia for individuals engaged in regular social interaction.[53] In addition, treatment and control of cognitive deficit in older patients may improve survival through better-enabled social interaction.[54]

The influence of parent–child relationships on geriatric well-being is most likely dependent on the nature of those relationships. Parents (aged 50–72 years) have been shown to demonstrate fewer depressive symptoms when relied upon by their adult children for instrumental support, such as chores, transportation, shopping, or financial aid. Expressive support of adult children, through life discussions or emotional encouragement, does not result in similar benefits.[55] This may be related to the general finding that older adults in "under-benefitted" relationships (giving more than they receive) or balanced relationships have fewer mental health disturbances than those receiving greater perceived benefit from others (unbalanced "over-benefitted" relationships).[56] Psychological distress is predicted for those receiving "too much" help or support from others, as this often indicates a relationship that is vulnerable to termination. Individuals involved in unbalanced relationships are particularly vulnerable to negative emotions in situations where there is decreased cultural support of longitudinal reciprocity (eg, "Senior parents deserve help and respect now because they took care of their children in the past"; "I help my spouse now because she has treated me well in the past").[57,58] Geriatric morbidity and mortality rates are lower in individuals who perceive themselves as useful to others.[59] Volunteering has been found to have greater positive impact on the subjective well-being of seniors than of younger individuals.[60]

Sexual Relationships

Most seniors believe that sexual activity is a vital part of life and important to the maintenance of good relationships.[61] Continued sexual functioning into advanced age has been associated with lower all-cause and stroke-specific mortality rates in both men and women.[62] The prevalence of sexual activity declines with advancing age, from 73% between age 57 and 64, to 53% in the 65- to 74-year-old age range. After age 74, prevalence drops to 26%. There is a positive correlation between general self-perception of health and extent of sexual undertaking. In all geriatric age groups, data reflect greater sexual activity among men than women. Nonsexual intimacy (eg, hugging, caressing) is quite common among seniors with partners (90% report frequent physical contact), and most seniors rate their relationships as physically and emotionally satisfying.[41] Approximately half of those sexually active report sexual problems, but only 30% of the geriatric population report having discussed their sex lives with a physician. The most common reported problems in women are decreased libido, inadequate lubrication, and inability to achieve climax. Erectile dysfunction is the most prevalent concern among men. Many complaints pertaining to sexual dysfunction are related to physical health issues, prompting some authors to recommend that older patients with a medical condition or treatment that carries implications for sexual function be counseled according to health rather than age.[63]

As is typical with younger individuals, a number of psychosocial factors can also inhibit sexual activity in seniors. The quality of the interpersonal relationship plays a significant role in sexual interest and enjoyment for couples of all ages, with relationship satisfaction predicting sexual satisfaction in all age groups.[64] Although seniors are no longer faced with barriers to sexual intimacy related to fertility, other issues of health and aging physical appearance may impact their comfort and willingness to engage in sexual activity. Many seniors may have incorrect perceptions about sexual norms and may be embarrassed to acknowledge ongoing sexual interest. Seniors may also experience feelings of guilt or shame when resuming sexual activity after the death of a spouse. An open and direct conversation initiated by a trusted physician can correct misconceptions, introduce medical supports for sexual activity, and serve as a forum to evaluate the need for specialized psychological treatment focused on sexual difficulties.

PSYCHOLOGICAL FACTORS

When it comes to staying young, a mind-lift beats a face-lift any day.

—Marty Bucella

Personality and Aging

Personality can be broadly defined as the cognitive, emotional, and behavioral tendencies that develop in childhood, through the interaction of temperament and social environment, and that remain fairly constant throughout the lifespan. When these tendencies change, they tend to do so gradually, over time, in response to alterations in an individual's social milieu.[65,66] Just as it has been demonstrated that a cluster of lifestyle behaviors (eg, poor diet, physical inactivity, tobacco use) are associated with a variety of health impacts (eg, cardiovascular risk, cancer), so also, there is emerging support[67–69] for the role of certain psychological tendencies ("the disease prone personality") and adverse aging outcomes, through their relationship to coping strategies, adherence to medical and preventive regimens, social relationships, and mental health.

The personality trait of "conscientiousness" is emerging as the cornerstone of the "self-healing personality" (healthy outcomes). Conscientiousness describes individuals who are "prudent, planful, persistent, and dependable."[68] Both childhood and mid-life conscientiousness are associated with decreased mortality risk. Prospective studies of elders have also shown a relationship between increased conscientiousness and improved longevity.[4,69] Conscientiousness has been shown to be positively associated with beneficial health behaviors and negatively associated with health risk behaviors, which may explain the mechanisms through which longevity is impacted.[70] Conscientious individuals are also likely to be well informed and adherent to medical recommendations.[71]

The ability to focus on positive emotions is also viewed as a protective psychological factor in the pursuit of optimal aging. For example, successful agers in the Nun Study have been the women scoring high in positive emotional expression (a tendency toward communication of positive feelings through verbal or nonverbal means) in early adulthood.[72] Other research using this sample (the members of the School Sisters of Notre Dame; participants in the "Nun Study") suggests longevity is associated with increased intellectual curiosity, a sense of thankfulness, and a strong connection to community.[73] Possessing a greater sense of purpose in life and a positive attitude about aging are also associated with successful aging (odds ratios .74–.99 and .90–.95, respectively).[11,74,75] Positive emotionality is thought to be related to beneficial physiological activity, which can buffer the impact of negative life events on the body.[51] These results are echoed in the common findings of enhanced longevity in optimistic individuals[76,77] and greater mortality in those high in negative affect[78] and neuroticism.[4] Fortunately, like many of the physical parameters that influence mortality (eg, blood pressure, cholesterol level), there are some indications that it is not only absolute level, but also trajectories of these traits that are important.[79] Despite the tendency to view personality characteristics as permanent, there is evidence that they change over time, through ongoing interactions of individual and environment.[80,81] This hints at the possibility that, through therapy or other effortful change, or significant change in social environment, individuals could decrease their levels of neuroticism, increase positive emotionality, and, possibly, achieve greater longevity.

Emotional Well-Being

Emotional well-being can be thought of as the balance a person experiences in positive and negative emotions. There is extensive evidence that emotional well-being improves in the decades between one's 30s and one's 60s.[14] Older age is associated with more pleasant emotional experiences (fewer negative emotions, sustained positive emotions)[82,83] and improved emotion regulation (decreased affective and physiological reactivity).[84,85]

Despite the reasonably good emotional adjustment enjoyed by most seniors, it is estimated that 6% to 23% of community-dwelling seniors experience depressive symptomatology.[86] Anxiety disorder prevalence rates are also significant (15%).[87] Both depression and anxiety have been found to increase mortality,[88] and depression strongly negatively correlates with successful aging.[89] There is, however, evidence that the increased morbidity and mortality associated with depression are short-lived effects, which can be normalized by psychological recovery.[90] Cognitive–behavioral (CBT) and behavioral therapies (BT) have been shown to be effective psychological interventions for depressed[91] and anxious[92] seniors.

Emotional well-being has also been associated with good sleep quality. Poor sleep has been associated with increased risk of major depression, memory problems, and fewer social interactions among seniors.[93,94] Despite the fact that seniors can achieve good sleep quality,[95] it is believed that 50% of older adults have significant problems with sleep onset or maintenance.[96] Good (restorative) sleep may be a marker for, or driver of, "successful aging." High-functioning seniors may sleep well, or sleeping well may actually support the ability of seniors to cope with challenges and remain socially engaged. Elderly individuals often have increased fall risk, making many sleep medications poor choices for insomnia treatment. Sleep hygiene education (which teaches patients about appropriate sleep habits) and sleep restriction procedures (which limit the amount of time in bed, discourage naps, and encourage strict sleep schedules) can be beneficial alternatives to medications. CBT for insomnia (which combines sleep hygiene and sleep restriction procedures with efforts to alter negative sleep-related cognitions) has been shown to be effective in older adults.[97]

Coping

Elders have increased vulnerability to physiological stressors (eg, extreme heat, cold, injury) due to age-related endocrine-, nervous-, and immune-system changes.[98] However, the degree to which elders are at increased risk in situations of psychological stress is unclear. Some chronic stressors are statistically more likely to confront older adults (eg, chronic illness, decreased financial resources, decreased social support due to death or disability of peers). Despite this fact, older adults tend to report fewer overall stressors and fewer daily hassles than younger adults. Older adults may also be less psychologically reactive to stressors,[99,100] commonly using coping strategies intended calm their emotions (rather than the problem-solving coping strategies favored by younger individuals) when challenged.[101] In addition, although the effectiveness of coping strategies is difficult to measure directly, older adults do perceive themselves as effective copers,[102] and there is little evidence of universal age-related declines in coping abilities.[103]

The most common acute stressors for seniors are interpersonal strains, financial/job changes, and health events.[104] Seniors rate health events as the most threatening and are most apt to use avoidance coping in response to this type of stressor. Individuals experiencing a greater total number of stressors are also more likely to use avoidance coping strategies, which are associated with greater depression and substance use.

One necessary skill for positive adaptation to chronic stressors is the ability to regulate one's emotions through seeking out and intentionally focusing on positive experiences, even during times of difficulty. This ability to have both positive and negative experiences during the same time period is known as "emotional complexity," which is associated with resilience to stressors.[105] It is believed that emotional complexity can be enhanced, both in seniors and in younger individuals, by Zen techniques such as the Mindfulness Meditation interventions pioneered by Jon Kabat-Zinn.[106,107]

Interventions to enhance coping skills are likely to have benefits for seniors across stressor domains.[104] Seniors challenged by significant stressors can also be assisted in positive coping by being encouraged to identify positive aspects of adverse events, engage in "active" (not avoidant) coping, and be more assertive.

Personal Autonomy/Control

"Sense of control" is a blanket term describing an individual's belief in his or her ability/efficacy to impact their environment. A strong sense of control is positively associated with longevity in the elderly.[108] Sense of control provides a resource individuals can draw upon as they confront the challenges of aging and, possibly, illness. A strong belief in the ability of one's actions to impact outcomes (internal locus of control) has been shown to be associated with greater subjective well-being, positive health behaviors (eg, exercise), improved adjustment to chronic illness, and less disease-related impairment. Coping strategies, among those with greater sense of control, are also more effective, which is important owing to the intractable nature of many late-life problems.

RELIGIOSITY AND SPIRITUALITY

To keep the heart unwrinkled, to be hopeful, kindly, cheerful, reverent—that is to triumph over old age.

—Thomas Bailey Aldrich

America is a highly religious nation, whether measured by belief (96% believe in a God or higher spirit) or practice (90% report praying regularly).[109] Recent age cohorts have demonstrated a tendency toward increased religiosity with age.[110] For example, the percentage of a population regularly attending church increases from young adulthood until physical health declines set in among the oldest-old.[111] Increased religiosity has been associated with decreased incidence of illness[112] (eg, cancer, heart disease, mental illness, high blood pressure), higher health-related quality of life, and decreased mortality, even after controlling for baseline health status and health behaviors.[113,114]

There has been extensive interest in how religion might impact morbidity and mortality. One demonstrable benefit of religiosity on health is the association between religious attendance and positive health behaviors, such as decreased use of tobacco and alcohol and increased exercise.[115] Conscientiousness, noted previously to be an important predictor of health, has been hypothesized to mediate the relationship between religiosity and health, underlying adherence to both religious mandates and preventive health recommendations.[116,117]

Prayer is one of the most common religious practices, and may facilitate health benefits on a number of levels. It has been shown that engaging in prayer elicits the relaxation response,[118] which can decrease blood pressure, heart rate, and metabolism. Praying for others may also allow seniors to feel they are helping, which has been shown, even in secular contexts, to provide health benefits.[119] Group prayer may also improve seniors' perceived social connectedness, reducing the loneliness some seniors experience. As noted earlier, social isolation has been associated with poor health outcomes.[120]

One of the primary benefits religiosity may offer for elders is a means of coping with the negative experiences of later life.[121] Seniors may turn to God (or any higher power) in positive ways (turning over problems, seeking guidance and strength), which buffers the impact of stressful life events on health. This form of coping may be especially useful for seniors owing to the nature of age-related stressors (health decline, mortality).[89] Religious worldviews may allow individuals to view stressful life and health events in ways that give meaning to their experiences, highlight the opportunities for growth through pain, or permit individuals to incorporate the negative event into a greater plan or purpose for their lives. Unfortunately, well-being can also be negatively impacted by an individual's religious beliefs. Seniors may experience increased anger and depression when confronted with events contradicting their notions of a just or loving God.[122] Several studies suggest increased mortality in patients who feel abandoned or punished by God while struggling with illness or recovery.[123,124]

Forgiveness is a major tenet of most religious traditions. Although there are many forms of forgiveness (forgiving self or others, asking for absolution from God or others), most research has focused on the health impacts of forgiving others. It has been shown that those who forgive others tend to have better mental health[125] and less anger and hostility,[126] which can decrease cardiovascular risk.[127,128]

In conclusion, the literature shows that meditation/relaxation strategies, social connection, and volunteerism are helpful and should be encouraged as possible health protective behaviors in all seniors. The research also suggests that teaching people to forgive (even in secular frameworks) may be useful.[129]

SUMMARY

Old age is like everything else. To make a success of it, you've got to start young.

—Theodore Roosevelt

This article has discussed a number of psychosocial factors associated with successful aging. Many of the derived recommendations cut across specific research domains, such as the importance of becoming and remaining socially integrated. Aging will be facilitated by maximizing contact with positive, supportive individuals and focusing on positive emotions, whenever possible. To make that possible, emotional, sexual, and sleep disturbances should be treated. Establishing personal habits such as regular meditation/relaxation practices, conscientiousness in pro-health behaviors, and volunteer work will also hold an individual in good stead throughout the lifespan. Finally, encouraging younger individuals to spend time with optimally aging seniors will allow for the development of positive aging attitudes, which will pay dividends in positive self-perceptions as those individuals age.

REFERENCES

1. Kirby SE, Coleman PG, Daley D. Spirituality and well-being in frail and nonfrail older adults. J Gerontol B Psychol Sci Soc Sci 2004;59(3):123–9.

2. U.S. Census Bureau. Annual projections of the resident population by age, sex, race, and Hispanic origin: lowest, middle, highest, and zero international migration series, 1999 to 2100. Available at: http://www.census.gov/population/www/projections/natdet.html. Accessed October 30, 2010.

3. Rowe JW, Kahn RL. Successful aging. New York: Pantheon Books; 1998.

4. Anderson NB, Armstead CA. Toward understanding the association of socioeconomic status and health: a new challenge for the biopsychosocial approach. Psychosom Med 1995;57(3):213–25.

5. Wilson RS, Mendes de Leon CF, Bienias JL, et al. Personality and mortality in old age. J Gerontol B Psychol Sci Soc Sci 2004;59(3):110–6.

6. Almeida OP, Norman P, Hankey G, et al. Successful mental health aging: results from a longitudinal study of older Australian men. Am J Geriatr Psychiatry 2006;14:27–35.

7. Vaillant GE, Mukamal K. Successful aging. Am J Psychiatry 2001;158(6):839–47.

8. House JS, Lepkowski JM, Kinney AM et al. The social stratification of aging and health. J Health Soc Behav 1994;35(3):213–34.

9. Yang Y. Long and happy living: trends and patterns of happy life expectancy in the U.S., 1970–2000. Soc Sci Res 2008;37(4):1235–52.

10. Jeste DV, Depp CA, Vahia IV. Successful cognitive and emotional aging. World Psychiatry 2010;9(2):78–84.

11. Silverstein S. The little boy and the old man In: A light in the attic. New York: HarperCollins; 1981.

12. Heckhausen J, Dickson RA, Baltes PB. Gains and losses in development throughout adulthood as perceived by different adult age groups. Dev Psychol 1989;25:109–21.

13. Perles T. Centenarians who avoid dementia. Trends Neurosci, 2004;27(10):633–6.

14. Federal Interagency Forum on Aging-Related Statistics. Older Americans 2010: Key Indicators of Well-Being. Available at: http://www.agingstats.gov/agingstatsdotnet/Main_Site/Data/2010_Documents/Docs/OA_2010.pdf. Accessed August 28, 2010.

15. Dunn ME. Psychological perspectives of sex and aging. Am J Cardiol 1988;61(16):24H–26H.

16. National Institute on Aging. The Health and Retirement Study: Growing Older in America, 2009. Available at: http://www.nia.nih.gov/. Accessed August 28, 2010.

17. Twenge JM, Catanese KR, Baumeister RF. Social exclusion causes self-defeating behaviors. J Pers Soc Psychol 2002;83:606–15.

18. Palmore EB. Ageism: negative and positive 2nd edition. New York: Springer Publishing; 1999.

19. Levy BR. Improving memory in old age by implicit self-stereotyping. J Pers Soc Psychol 1996;71:1092–107.

20. Hess TM, Hinson JT, Statham JA. Implicit and explicit stereotype activation effects on memory: Do age and awareness moderate the impact of priming? Psychol Aging 2004;19:495–505.

21. Goldman R, Goldman G. How children view old people and aging: a developmental study of children in four countries. Austral J Psychol 1981;33:405–18.

22. O'Hanlon AM, Camp CJ, Osofsky HJ. Knowledge of and attitudes toward aging in young, middle aged and older collge students. Educ Gerontol 1993;19:753–66.

23. Ron P. Elderly people's attitudes and perceptions of aging and old age: the role of cognitive dissonance? Int J Geriatr Psychiatry 2007;22:656–62.

24. Kaufman SR. The ageless self: sources of meaning in late life. Madison (WI): University of Wisconsin Press; 1987.

25. Davis NC, Friedrich D. Age stereotypes in middle-aged through old-old adults. Int J Aging Hum Dev 2010;70(3):199–212.

26. Levy BR, Slade MD, Kasl SV. Longitudinal benefit of positive self-perceptions of aging on functional health. J Gerontol B Psychol Sci Soc Sci 2002;57:409–17.

27. Levy BR, Myers MM. Preventive health behaviors influenced by self-perceptions of aging. Prev Med 2004;39:625–9.

28. Wrosch C, Bauer I, Miller GE, et al. Regret intensity, diurnal cortisol secretion, and physical health in older individuals: evidence for directional effects and protective factors. Psychol Aging 2007;22:319–30.

29. Greene MG, Adelman RD, Charon R, et al. Concordance between physicians and their older and younger patients in primary care medical encounters. Gerontologist 1989;29:808–13.

30. Derby SE. Ageism in cancer care of the elderly. Oncol Nurs Forum 1991;18:921–6.

31. Ory M, Hoffman MK, Hawkins M, et al. Challenging aging stereotypes: strategies for creating a more active society. Am J Prev Med 2003;25(3Sii):164–71.

32. Hess TM. Attitudes toward aging. In: Birren JE, Schaie KW, editors. Handbook of the psychology of aging. 6th edition. Burlington (MA): Elsevier; 2006. p. 379–406.

33. Carstensen LL, Isaacowitz DM, Charles ST. Taking time seriously: a theory of socioemotional selectivity. Am Psychol 1999;54(3):165–81.

34. Mather M, Carstensen LL. Aging and motivated cognition: the positivity effect in attention and memory. Trends Cogn Sci 2005;9(10):496–502.

35. Kliegel M, Jäger T, Phillips LH. Emotional development across adulthood: differential age-related emotional reactivity and emotion regulation in a negative mood induction procedure. Int J Aging Hum Dev 2007;64(3):217–44.

36. Knight BG, Maines ML, Robinson GS. The effects of sad mood on memory in older adults: a test of the mood congruence effect. Psychol Aging 2002;17(4):653–61.

37. Segal DL, Needham TN, Coolidge FL. Age differences in attachment orientations among younger and older adults: evidence from two self-report measures of attachment. Int J Aging Hum Dev 2009;69(2):119–32.

38. Hendricks J, Cutler SJ. Volunteerism and socioemotional selectivity in later life. J Gerontol B Psychol Sci Soc Sci 2004;59(5):S251–7.

39. Ersner-Hershfield H, Mikels JA, Sullivan SJ, et al. Poignancy: mixed emotional experience in the face of meaningful endings. J Pers Soc Psychol 2008;94(1):158–67.

40. Seeman TE, Crimmins E. Social environment effects on health and aging: integrating epidemiologic and demographic approaches and perspectives. Ann NY Acad Sci 2001;954:88–117.

41. Helgeson VS, Cohen S, Fritz HL. Social ties and cancer. In: Holland JC, Breitbart W, editors. Psycho-oncology. New York: Oxford Press; 1998. p. 99–109.

42. Cohen S, Doyle WJ, Skoner DP, et al. Social ties and susceptibility to the common cold. JAMA 1997;277(24):1940–4.

43. Rutledge T, Linke SE, Olson MB, et al. Social networks and incident stroke among women with suspected myocardial ischemia. Psychosom Med 2008;70(3):282–97.

44. Kop WJ, Berman DS, Gransar H, et al. Social network and coronary artery calcification in asymptomatic individuals. Psychosom Med 2005;67(3):343–52.

45. Rutledge T, Reis SE, Olson M, et al. Social networks are associated with lower mortality rates among women with suspected coronary artery disease: The National Heart, Lung, and Blood Institute–sponsored Women's Ischemia Syndrome Evaluation Study. Psychosom Med 2004;66(6):882–8.

46. Seeman TE, Crimmins E. Social environment effects on health and aging: integrating epidemiologic and demographic approaches and perspectives. Ann NY Acad Sci 2001;954:88–117.

47. Charles ST, Carstensen LL. Social and emotional aging. Annu Rev Psychol 2010; 61:383–409.

48. Rowe JL, Conwell Y, Shulberg HC, et al. Social support and suicidal ideation in older adults using home healthcare services. Am J Geriatr Psychiatry 2006;14(9):758–66.
49. House JS, Landis KR, Umberson D. Social relationships and health. Science 1988;241(4865):540–5.
50. Rook KS. The negative side of social interactions: impact on psychological well-being. J Pers Soc Psychol 1984;46(5):1097–108.
51. Burns R, Nichols LO, Graney MJ, et al. Impact of continued geriatric outpatient management on health outcomes of older veterans. Arch Intern Med 1995;155(12): 1313–8.
52. Pitkala KH, Routasalo P, Kautiainen H, et al. Effects of psychosocial group rehabilitation on health, use of health care services, and mortality of older persons suffering from loneliness: a randomized, controlled trial. J Gerontol A Biol Sci Med Sci 2009;64(7):792–800.
53. Wang HX, Karp A, Winblad B, et al. Late-life engagement in social and leisure activities is associated with a decreased risk of dementia: a longitudinal study from the Kungsholmen project. Am J Epidemiol 2002;155(12):1081–7.
54. Sampson EL, Bulpitt CJ, Fletcher AE. Survival of community-dwelling older people: the effect of cognitive impairment and social engagement. J Am Geriatr Soc 2009;57(6):985–91.
55. Byers AL, Levy BR, Allore HG, et al. When parents matter to their adult children: filial reliance associated with parents' depressive symptoms. J Gerontol B Psychol Sci Soc Sci 2008;63(1):33–40.
56. Fyrand L. Reciprocity: a predictor of mental health and continuity in elderly people's relationships? A review. Curr Gerontol Geriatr Res 2010; pii: 340161.
57. Antonucci TC, Akiyama H. Social networks in adult life and a preliminary examination of the convoy model. J Gerontol 1987;42(5):519–27.
58. Neufeld A, Harrison MJ. Men as caregivers: reciprocal relationships or obligation? J Adv Nurs 1998;28(5):959–68.
59. Gruenewald TL, Karlamangla AS, Greendale GA, et al. Feelings of usefulness to others, disability, and mortality in older adults: the MacArthur study of successful aging. J Gerontol B Psychol Sci Soc Sci 2007;62(1):28–37.
60. Van Willigen M. Differential benefits of volunteering across the life course. J Gerontol B Psychol Sci Soc Sci 2000;55(5):308–18.
61. Waite LJ, Laumann, EO, Das A, et al. Sexuality: measures of partnerships, practices, attitudes and problems in the National Social Life, Health, and Aging Study. J Gerontol B Psychol Sci Soc Sci 2009;64(1):i56–66.
62. Chen HK, Tseng CD, Wu SC. A prospective cohort study on the effect of sexual activity, libido, and widowhood on mortality among the elderly people: 14 year follow-up of 2453 elderly Taiwanese. Int J Epidemiol 2007;36(5):1136–42.
63. Lindau ST, Schumm LP, Laumann EO, et al. A study of sexuality and health among older adults in the United States. N Engl J Med 2007;357(8):762–74.
64. Meston C. Aging and sexuality. West J Med 1997;167(4):285–90.
65. Caspi A, Roberts BW, Shiner RL. Personality development: stability and change. Annu Rev Psychol 2005;56:453–84.
66. Ardelt M. Still stable after all these years? Personality stability theory revisted. Soc Psychol Q 2000;63(4):392–405.
67. Terracciano A, Lockenhoff CE, Zonderman AB, et al. Personality predictors of longevity: activity, emotional stability, and conscientiousness. Psychosom Med 2008;70(6):621–7.

68. Friedman HS, Martin LR. A lifespan approach to personality and longevity: the case of conscientiousness. In: Aldwin CM, Park CL, Spiro A, editors. Handbook of health psychology and aging. New York: Guilford; 2007. p. 167–85.

69. Weiss A, Costa PT. Domain and facet personality predictors of all-cause mortality among Medicare patients aged 65–100. Psychosom Med 2005;67(5):724–33.

70. Bogg T, Roberts BW. Conscientiousness and health-related behaviors: a meta-analysis of the leading behavioral contributors to mortality. Psychol Bull 2004;130(6):887–919.

71. Christensen AJ, Smith TW. Personality and patient adherence: correlates of the five-factor model in renal dialysis. J Behav Med 1995;18(3):305–13.

72. Danner DD, Snowdon DA, Friesen WV. Positive emotions in early life and longevity: findings from the Nun Study. J Pers Soc Psychol 2001;80(5):804–13.

73. Snowdon D. Aging with grace: what the Nun Study teaches us about leading longer, healthier, and more meaningful lives. New York: Bantam Books; 2001.

74. Andrews GJ, Clark M, Luszcz M. Successful aging in the Australian Longitudinal Study of Aging: applying the MacArthur model cross-nationally. J Soc Issues 2002;4:749–65.

75. Krause N. Meaning in life and mortality. J Gerontol B Psychol Sci Soc Sci 2009;64(4): 517–27.

76. Maruta T, Colligan RC, Malinchoc M, et al. Optimists vs pessimists: survival rate among medical patients over a 30-year period. Mayo Clin Proc 2000;75(2):140–3.

77. Giltay EJ, Geleijnse JM, Zitman FG, et al. Dispositional optimism and all-cause and cardiovascular mortality in a prospective cohort of elderly Dutch men and women. Arch Gen Psychiatry 2004;61:1126–35.

78. Wilson RS, Bienias JL, Mendes de Leon CF, et al. Negative affect and mortality in older persons. Am J Epidemiol 2003;158(9):827–35.

79. Mroczek DK, Spiro A. Personality change influences mortality in older men. Psychol Sci 2007;18(5):371–6.

80. Mroczek DK, Spiro A. Modeling intraindividual change in personality traits: findings from the Normative Aging Study. J Gerontol B Psychol Sci Soc Sci 2003;58(3):153–65.

81. Hooker K, McAdams DP. Personality reconsidered: a new agenda for aging research. J Gerontol B Psychol Sci Soc Sci 2003;58(6):296–304.

82. Carstensen LL, Fung H, Charles S. Socioemotional selectivity theory and the regulation of emotion in the second half of life. Motiv Emotion 2003;27(2):102–23.

83. Carstensen LL, Pasupathi M, Mayr U, et al. Emotional experience in everyday life across the adult life span. J Pers Soc Psychol 2000;79(4):644–55.

84. Charles ST, Piazza JR, Luong G, et al. Now you see it, now you don't; age differences in affective reactivity to social tensions. Psychol Aging 2009;24(3):645–53.

85. Levenson RW. Expressive, physiological, and subjective changes in emotion across adulthood. In: Qualls SH, Abeles N, editors. Psychology and the aging revolution: how we adapt to longer life. Washington, DC: American Psychological Association; 2000. p. 123–40.

86. Gallo JJ, Lebowitz BD. The epidemiology of common late-life mental disorders in the community: themes for the new century. Psychiatr Serv 1999;50(9):1158–66.

87. Mehta KM, Simonsick EM, Penninx BW, et al. Prevalence and correlates of anxiety symptoms in well-functioning older adults: findings from the Health Aging and Body Composition Study. J Am Geriatr Soc 2003;51(4):499–504.

88. Tennant C, McLean L. The impact of emotions on coronary heart disease risk. J Cardiovasc Risk 2001;8(3):175–83.

89. Depp CA, Jeste DV. Definitions and predictors of successful aging: a comprehensive review of larger quantitative studies. Am J Geriatr Psychiatr 2006;14(1):6–20.

90. Lesperance F, Frasure-Smith N, Talajic M, et al. Five-year risk of cardiac mortality in relation to initial severity and one-year changes in depression symptoms after myocardial infarction. Circulation 2002;105(5):1049–53.

91. Pinquart M, Sorensen S. How effective are psychotherapeutic and other psychosocial interventions with older adults? A meta-analysis. J Ment Health Aging 2001;7: 207–43.

92. Wetherell JL, Gatz M, Craske MG. Treatment of generalized anxiety disorder in older adults. J Consult Clin Psychol 2003;71(1):31–40.

93. Walsh JK. Clinical and socioeconomic correlates of insomnia. J Clin Psychiatr 2004; 65(Suppl 8):13–9.

94. Dew MA, Reynolds CF, Monk TH, et al. Psychosocial correlates and sequelae of electroencephalographic sleep in healthy elders. J Gerontol 1994;49:8–18.

95. Driscoll HC, Serody L, Patrick S, et al. Sleeping well, aging well: a descriptive and cross-sectional study of sleep in "successful agers" 75 and older. Am J Geriatr Psychiatry 2008;16(1):74–82.

96. Foley DJ, Monjan AA, Brown SL, et al. Sleep complaints among elderly persons: an epidemiologic study of three communities. Sleep 1995;18(6):425–32.

97. Pallesen S, Nordhus I, Kvale G. Nonpharmacological interventions for insomnia in older adults: a meta-analysis of treatment efficacy. Psychotherapy 1998;35:472–82.

98. Aldwin CM, Gilmer DF. Health, illness, and optimal aging: biological and psychosocial perspectives. Thousand Oaks (CA): SAGE; 2004.

99. Johnson NJ, Backlund E, Sorlie PD, et al. Marital status and mortality: the national longitudinal mortality study. Ann Epidemiol 2000;10(4):224–38.

100. Park CL, Aldwin CM, Fenster JR, et al. Pathways to post-traumatic growth versus post-traumatic stress: coping and emotional reactions following the September 11, 2001 terrorist attacks. Am J Orthopsychiatry 2008;78(3):300–12.

101. Rothermund K, Brandtstäder J. Coping with deficits and losses in later life: from compensatory action to accommodation. Psychol Aging 2003;18(4):896–905.

102. Aldwin CM, Sutton KJ, Chiara G, Spiro A. Age differences in stress, coping, and appraisal: findings from the normative aging study. J Gerontol B Psychol Sci Soc Sci 1996;51(4):179–88.

103. Aldwin CM, Yancura LA, Boeninger DK. Coping, health, and aging. In: Aldwin CM, Park CL, Spiro A, editors. Handbook of health psychology and aging. New York: Guilford; 2007. p. 210–26.

104. Moos RH, Brennan PL, Schutte KK, et al. Older adults' coping with negative life events: common processes of managing health, interpersonal, and financial/work stressors. In J Aging Hum Dev 2006;62(1):39–59.

105. Davis MC, Zautura AJ, Johnson LM, et al. Psychosocial stress, emotion regulation, and resilience among older adults. In: Aldwin CM, Park CL, Spiro A, editors. Handbook of health psychology and aging. New York: Guilford; 2007. p. 250–66.

106. Kabat-Zinn J. Wherever you go, there go, there you are: mindfulness meditation in everyday life. New York: Hyperion; 1994.

107. Kabat-Zinn J, Lipworth L, Burney R. The clinical use of mindfulness meditation for the self-regulation of chronic pain. J Behav Med 1985;8(2):163–90.

108. Skaff MM. Sense of control and health: dynamic duo in the aging process. In: Aldwin CM, Park CL, Spiro A, editors. Handbook of health psychology and aging. New York: Guilford; 2007. p. 186–209.

109. Gallup Organization. Focus on religion. Available at: http://www.gallup.com/poll/14446/update-americans-religion.aspx. Accessed October 20, 2010.

110. Krause N. Religion and health in late life. In: Birren JE, Schaie KW, editors. Handbook of the psychology of Aging. 6th edition. Burlington (MA) Elsevier; 2006. p. 499–518.

111. Koenig HG, McCullough ME, Larson DB. Handbook of religion and health. New York: Oxford University Press; 2001.

112. George LK, Ellison CG, Larson BD. Explaining the relationship between religious involvement and health. Psychol Inquiry 2002;13:190–200.

113. Oman D, Kurata JH, Strawbridge WJ. Religious attendance and cause of death over 31 years. Int J Psychiatry Med 2002;32(1):69–89.

114. Thoreson CE, Harris AHS. Spirituality and health: What's the evidence and what's needed? Ann Behav Med 2002;24:3–13.

115. Strawbridge WJ, Cohen RD, Shema SJ. Frequent attendance at religious services and mortality over 28 years. Am J Public Health 1997;87:957–61.

116. Piedmont RL. The role of personality in understanding religious and spiritual constructs. In: Paloutzian RF, Park CL, editors. Handbook of the psychology of religion and spirituality. New York: Guilford; 2005. p. 253–73.

117. Reindl Benjamins M, Brown C. Religion and preventive health care utilization among the elderly. Soc Sci Med 2004;58:109–18.

118. Benson H. Timeless healing: the power and biology of belief. New York: Scribner; 1996.

119. Krause N. Church-based social support and health in old age: exploring variations by race. J Gerontol B Psychol Sci Soc Sci 2003;57:96–107.

120. Cohen S. Social relationships and health. Am Psychologist 2004;59:676–84.

121. Pergamet KI. The psychology of religion and coping: theory, research, and practice. New York: Guilford; 1997.

122. Exline JJ, Rose E. Religious and spiritual struggles. In: Paloutzian RF, Park CL, editors. The handbook of the psychology of religion and spirituality. New York: Guilford; 2005. p. 315–30.

123. Pergament KI, Koenig HG, Tarakeshwar N, et al. Religious struggle as a predictor of mortality among medically ill elderly patients: a 2-year longitudinal study. Arch Intern Med 2001;61:1881–5.

124. Oxman TE, Freeman DH, Manheimer ED. Lack of social participation or religious strength and comfort as risk factors for death after cardiac surgery in the elderly. Psychosom Med 1995;57:5–15.

125. Thoreson CE, Harris AH, Luskin F. Forgiveness and health: an unanswered question. In: McCullough ME, Pargament KI, Thoreson CE, editors. Forgiveness: theory, research, and practice. New York: Guildford; 2000. p. 254–80.

126. Bono G, McCullough ME. Religion, forgiveness, and adjustment in older adulthood. In: Schaie KW, Krause N, Booth A, editors. Religious influence on health and well-being in the elderly. New York: Springer; 2004. p. 163–86.

127. Williams JE. Anger/hostility and cardiovascular disease. In: Potegal M, Stemmler G, Spielberger C, editors. International handbook of anger: constituent and concomitant biological, psychological, and social processes. New York: Springer; p. 435–47.

128. Smith TW, Glazer K, Ruiz JM. Hostility, anger, aggressiveness, and coronary heart disease: an interpersonal perspective on personality, emotion, and health. J Pers 2004;72(6):1217–70.

129. Hargrave TD, Anderson WT. Finishing well: aging and reparation in the intergenerational family. New York: Bruner/Mazel; 1992.

Aging and Exercise

Jeralyn Allen, MD*, Vincent Morelli, MD

KEYWORDS
- Elderly • Exercise • Benefits • Barriers

Aging is a complex process that involves the interaction of both physiologic and behavioral factors. Generally, as people grow older, the basal metabolic rate slows; blood pressure increases; and there is a decrease in maximum heart rate, cardiac output, maximal oxygen consumption, and overall muscle mass. Other changes that can occur include a decline in cognitive function, reduced lung compliance, and decreased bone mass.

Not only does exercise ameliorate these changes of aging, but it also helps ward off modern-day "sedentary diseases" such as coronary artery disease (CAD), diabetes, hypertension, and osteoporosis[1–3] that contribute to premature aging and death.

Approximately 60% of adults do not exercise regularly and approximately 31% are completely sedentary. Activity levels tend to decrease with age, especially in adults 65 years of age and older, and 50% of this population have no plan to initiate an exercise program.[4,5] The groups who have an increased likelihood of exhibiting sedentary behavior include those of advanced age, female gender, nonwhite ethnicity, lower educational levels, and lower income.[6]

This article discusses the benefits of exercise in the elderly and how physicians can help such patients overcome barriers to exercise (eg, lack of education, coexisting morbidities), and also offers some practical exercise prescriptions for both healthy and compromised elderly patients.

BENEFITS

Numerous benefits to exercising have long been proven. Cardiovascular improvements are seen in the form of physiologic parameters (eg, $\dot{V}o_2$max, cardiac output), improvement in blood pressure, decreased risk of CAD, improvements in congestive heart failure (CHF), and improvement in lipid profiles.[7–10]

The incidence of type 2 diabetes mellitus is decreased among patients who exercise.[11] For those who already have the diagnosis, exercise improves glycemic control, decreases hemoglobin A1C levels, and improves insulin sensitivity.[12] Benefits also include improvements in bone health. Exercise lessens bone loss in postmenopausal women,

Department of Family and Community Medicine, Meharry Medical College, 1005 Dr D. B. Todd, Jr, Boulevard, Nashville, TN 37208, USA
* Corresponding author.
E-mail address: jeralyn_allen@yahoo.com

Clin Geriatr Med 27 (2011) 661–671
doi:10.1016/j.cger.2011.07.010
0749-0690/11/$ – see front matter © 2011 Elsevier Inc. All rights reserved.

decreases hip and vertebral fractures, decreases risk of falls, and improves joint function by decreasing pain in arthritic patients.[13]

Exercise also provides neuropsychological health benefits. It improves sleep quality and cognitive function and decreases rates of depression.[14,15] In addition, exercise decreases the incidence of colon and breast cancer[16–18] and decreases all-cause morbidity and mortality.[19]

There is increasing interest in the area of exercise and its effect on longevity. In rodents, exercise has been found to improve health but not longevity. In humans, there is some evidence that exercise increases longevity,[20,21] but this is based on retrospective data, not on high-quality prospective trials.

BARRIERS TO EXERCISE

Lack of physical activity is an increasing public health concern[22] that is not excluded in the elderly population. Pain and concerns about poor health are the two most common barriers to exercise in the elderly.[23] Other barriers include inadequate physician education, patient myths concerning exercise, as well as social and environmental factors. Many elderly patients view exercise as "too time consuming," noting that transit time to exercise facilities as well as time spent exercising are non-motivators.[24] The physical environment in which one lives can be a factor. The availability of exercise facilities or convenience of resources for exercise, as well as crime level in the environment, may influence level of activity.[25] Primary care physicians should help patients overcome these barriers and move toward a healthier lifestyle through focused patient education and the design of an achievable exercise program.

EDUCATING SENIORS ABOUT BENEFITS AND BARRIERS

Clinicians play a significant role in the promotion of exercise. As people age, the frequency of physician visits increases,[26] and these visits provide opportunities to educate and motivate. Studies have shown that direct physician counseling is the most effective means of influencing patient behavior in terms of exercise promotion.[27]

Safety

For an older person, safety is a major concern when starting an exercise program. Approximately one out of three adults older than 65 years reports falls each year,[28] so fall prevention is an important issue to address in the initiation and maintenance of an exercise regimen. People who previously experienced falls, whether or not injury was involved, may develop a fear or falling and, as a result, limit their activities, which may lead to a reduction in physical activity.[29]

Once a patient has fallen, it is important to evaluate the cause of the fall. In the outpatient setting, this includes careful history-taking, scrutiny of medications, evaluation of the many risk factors for falling, and a physical examination to include evaluation of postural control and physical ability.[30] The one-leg balance test is one such "fall prevention" screening exam. In this test, the patient stands on one leg without assistance, while flexing the opposite knee. The goal is for the patient to stand for 5 seconds in this position.[31] Inability to complete this test calls for strengthening programs to be included in the exercise regimen (as discussed later). Another important test is the "get up and go test." A patient is asked to rise from a standard armchair, walk a distance of 10 feet, then turn, walk back to the chair, and return to a seated position. Patients may use walking aids, but otherwise are unassisted. A test time of 30 seconds or greater is indicative of impaired mobility.[32] In older adults with balance issues, Tai chi and physical therapy also have been shown to be beneficial in preventing falls.[33] In addition, it is important to determine if medications and the home environment are safe. Drug side effects or polypharmacy may contribute to fall risk; thus, medication review is an important part of a pre-exercise evaluation.

Treat Comorbidities

Comorbid medical or psychiatric conditions should not be thought of as contraindications to exercise. In fact, physical activity has been shown to be associated with improvements in many of these conditions.[14,34] However, it is important to optimize treatment of comorbid medical conditions before beginning exercise programs. In addition, primary care physicians should periodically monitor patients in hopes of increasing exercise compliance and, perhaps, decreasing medication dosages as these chronic conditions improve. It is also important to screen regularly for deterioration in vision to optimize vision for physical activities.

Tools to Motivate

An exercise program should include gradual activity progression with achievable short-term goals. An individual's belief in his or her ability to exercise can be a determinant of how active or inactive he or she will be. The stronger people's expectations and perceived successes, the more likely they will initiate and continue with exercise.[24] Discussions with patients are opportunities to set short- and long-term goals. Counseling patients on the expected functional gains from increased strength and aerobic capacity can increase compliance.[35,36] Feelings of pleasure and satisfaction and a regular monitoring of patient progress are some of the most important factors in exercise prescription adherence.[24]

In the green prescription study,[37] sedentary patients given written exercise instructions were more compliant that those given only verbal instructions. Thus, the prescription pad can serve as a motivational tool when combined with active physician counseling.[38]

Several studies have examined how best to motivate seniors to *continue* compliance with exercise regimens.[27,39–43] Several of these studies have found motivational office visits, in which the importance of exercise was stressed by health care providers, useful in maintaining increased physical activity in elderly participants in the short but not long term.[42–45]

However, the most recent data *have* demonstrated some continued long-term adherence (up to 1 year) to exercise prescriptions with follow-up health provider contact or computer-generated telephone reminders.[46] In addition, when counseling patients, it is beneficial for physicians to be familiar with the accessibility of community facilities and organized health programs within the patient's community. The elderly are more likely to change their level of activity if time is spent counseling and providing information on specific companies or agencies that offer exercise programs.[47] Together with offering knowledge of where to go for exercise, providing a level of socialization begets success.[48] Organized physical activity can motivate elders to continue an exercise regimen. Especially in elderly women, a higher level of exercise compliance is associated with social support.[49]

EXERCISE SCREENING

Pre-participation screening is important in maintaining patient safety and determining the level at which intensity physical activity can begin. A thorough history and physical examination should be performed to stratify patients and identify physical limitations and concerning symptoms.

Absolute contraindications for exercise in the elderly are generally related to cardiac conditions and include acute coronary syndrome, third-degree AV block, uncontrolled hypertension, and *acute* heart failure. In addition, uncontrolled diabetes is an absolute contraindication due to lack of normal glucoregulation.

Relative contraindications include cardiomyopathy, valvular heart disease, and complex ventricular ectopy. Those with relative contraindications should still participate in exercise, but at a lower level of intensity and after careful medical evaluation. Patients with known CAD, symptoms of CAD, multiple cardiac risk factors, suspected diabetes, or known or suspected lung disease should undergo stress testing before starting an exercise program.[50]

Cardiac stress testing is also recommended for those with known CAD, two or more cardiac risk factors, diabetes, or major signs/symptoms of pulmonary or significant metabolic disease. In addition, men older than 45 and women older than 55 years of age who want to begin a *vigorous* exercise regimen ($>60\%$ $\dot{V}o_2$max) should undergo stress testing before initiation.

EXERCISE PRESCRIPTION

The recommended levels of activity for elderly patients should include a combination of aerobic exercise, strength training, flexibility, and balance exercises. According to the American College of Sports Medicine, in an update developed by a panel of experts, it is recommended that patients adhere to the following regimen:

1. Frequency: Exercise most days of the week.
2. Duration: 20 to 60 minutes of continuous or intermittent aerobic exercise. Activities of lower intensity should be performed for a longer duration (at least 30 minutes) whereas those of higher intensity can be done in shorter bouts.
3. Intensity: Physically fit patients should exercise at approximately 60% to 90% of maximal heart rate (206.9 − [0.67 × age]), or 50% to 85% of oxygen uptake reserve (the difference between maximal and resting $\dot{V}o_2$). Patients who are not physically fit should begin at an intensity of 55% to 64% of maximal heart rate and 40% to 49% of $\dot{V}o_2$max.
4. Mode: Use of large muscle groups in a continuous aerobic fashion is the goal of exercise, for example, walking, hiking, jogging, and swimming.
5. Resistance training: This is important in enhancing strength and preventing falls. It is recommended that patients participate in two to three sessions per week. One to three sets of eight to ten exercises targeted at major muscle groups should be done.[51]

Patients should be counseled on the level of intensity they should use during exercise. A low intensity level allows for talking or singing, muscles feel normal, and there is no perspiration. Moderate intensity allows for talking but not singing, perspiration but normal muscle feeling. High intensity does not allow for easy talking and muscles feel some fatigue. It is important that most patients begin at a moderate level of exercise if no other risk factors exist. In those who need a graduated exercise program, beginning at a low intensity and working up to moderate is best.

Aerobic Programs

Aerobic programs for the elderly should correspond to the patient's needs and abilities. Excellent examples include walking briskly, jogging, running, swimming, cycling, tennis, and golfing without a golf cart. If the patient is new to exercise, it is best to start with 5 to 10 minutes of cardiovascular exercises three times a week, allowing the patient to become acclimated. Patients may be graduated up to continuous aerobic activity for 30 or more minutes most days of the week. Always stress the importance of a warm-up with 5 or more minutes of light activity and stretching after the workout.

Resistance Programs

Major muscle groups should be included in resistance programs, to include chest, back, shoulders, arms, abdomen, and legs. Resistance bands are an excellent tool for seniors because they offer a safe alternative to the use of heavier free weights. Choose a band that offers a medium resistance. Specific exercises include the following:

Knee extensions

Have the patient sit in a chair and tie a loose loop around one ankle with a resistance band. The other end of the band should be secured around a leg of the chair. Have the patient slowly raise and straighten the leg in question. He or she will then lower the leg and repeat the motion for 10 to 15 repetitions on each side. As the exercise gets easier, have the patient progress to two sets of 10 to 15 repetitions.

Ankle flexion

Have the patient sit on the ground with both legs straight out in front. Tie one end of the resistance band around the toe and the other end to a sturdy object positioned level with the ankle in front. Using the hands for support, slowly flex and extend the ankle. Repeat 10 to 15 times on each side and increase repetitions as strength is built.

Bicep curl

Have the patient sit on a chair with the back straight and shoulders relaxed. Take one end of the band in each hand and place the feet on the band to keep it on the ground. Bend the elbows up so the hands approach the shoulders, then lower them to the starting position. Repeat this exercise 10 to 15 times and increase sets as strength increases.

Seated row

Have the patient sit in a chair and hold the ends of a resistance band in each hand. Place the feet on the middle of the band, holding the band to the floor. Have the patient start with hands and arms beside the legs. Then, slowly pull both elbows up and back, then return them to the starting position, as if to pull the bands backward. Repeat this exercise 10 to 15 times and progress as tolerated.

Balance Program

Balance exercises can be incorporated by adding an exercise ball. As an aid to balance, the ball can be used in place of a chair. Another balance exercise is the single-leg stand. The patient begins by standing on one foot while stabilizing him- or herself lightly, resting a hand on a chair or wall for 10 seconds and then alternating feet. Another exercise is the staggered stance. Here, the patient steps forward with one foot, maintains this position for 10 seconds, then repeats with the opposite foot. It is important that the patient lift his or her chest and keep his or her gaze locked on the wall at eye level.

Flexibility Program

Flexibility is important for exercise safety. Stretching may produce a mild pulling sensation, but should not cause pain. Patients should be instructed not to bounce into stretches, but instead gradually stretch into each movement. Several stretching programs are easily available on the Internet and, generally, 10 to 30 seconds of stretching is maintained before returning to neutral position. Stretches are repeated three to five times.[52]

SPECIAL CONSIDERATIONS
Dementia

There is evidence that exercise delays the onset of Alzheimer's dementia (AD),[53–56] reduces the incidence of the disease,[57] and reduces age-related brain function loss. In one study,[53] it was shown that those who exercised three or more times per week were more likely to be dementia free than those who exercised less frequently.

Patients who already have a diagnosis of AD have also been shown to benefit from exercise. A recent meta-analysis of more than 2000 patients with AD demonstrated that exercise resulted in significant increases in strength and flexibility and decreased behavioral, functional, and cognitive deficits.[57,58] Patients with AD can adhere to the same exercise guidelines as their nondemented counterparts, but with closer monitoring.

Osteoarthritis

Both aerobic exercise and resistance training have been shown to decrease disability and improve painful symptoms in patients with osteoarthritis (OA).[13] However, because an increased risk of knee pain and further joint damage exists in patients with quadriceps weakness, primary care physicians should include quadriceps strengthening exercises (to reduce the load on the knees) in their exercise prescriptions for patients with OA.[59,60]

Chronic Obstructive Pulmonary Disease

Patients with chronic obstructive pulmonary disease (COPD) also benefit from exercise. Endurance exercise is extremely important in these patients. According to The American Thoracic Society, a patient with a forced expiratory volume in 1 second (FEV$_1$) less than 50% to 60% should be considered for pulmonary rehabilitation.[61]

Pulmonary rehabilitation programs should aim for patients to exercise 3 to 5 days per week for at least 20 to 40 minutes. For resistance training, one to three sets of eight to twelve exercises, two to three times per week is recommended.[62] Pulmonary rehabilitation benefits patients with known COPD by increasing patients' walking endurance, reducing mortality and morbidity (thereby reducing hospital admissions), and improving health-related quality of life.[63] The goals of pulmonary rehabilitation are to reduce COPD symptoms and disability, improve quality of life in terms of independence, and increase social and physical participation. Outpatient rehabilitation programs are normally attended two to three times per week for 6 to 8 weeks and need to be continued indefinitely. Techniques learned involve strengthening respiratory muscles (to decrease fatigue when being active), pursed lip breathing, and pulmonary hygiene.

Congestive Heart Failure

There is no consensus on an exact regimen that patients with congestive heart failure (CHF) should follow. These patients should receive individualized prescriptions. In Class II to III CHF patients with less than 40% ejection fraction (EF), aerobic exercise has been shown to increase exercise tolerance and $\dot{V}o_2$max by 12% to 33%.[64] In addition, there is evidence that, along with adherence to a medication regimen, aerobic exercise can decrease mortality and the number of repeat hospitalizations. Strength training in this group produced up to a 43% increase in strength and a 13% increase in 6-minute walk distance.[64] Gradual and graded exercise programs are best for these patients, beginning with simple strength and resistance training and gradually increasing intensity to include more aerobic exercises as the patient improves and can tolerate it.

Hypertension

According to the Framingham Heart Study, 90% of people who are normotensive at age 55 years will eventually develop hypertension. Hypertension increases the risk for end-organ damage, coronary events, stroke, heart failure, and peripheral vascular disease.[65,66]

With normal aging, there is decreased arterial compliance and an increase in sympathetic tone. Exercise is beneficial because it improves these parameters; it increases arterial elasticity and decreases sympathetic tone, resulting in decreased blood pressure. Exercise can improve blood pressure by roughly 10/7 mm Hg. Hypertensive patients should participate in approximately 30 minutes of moderate intensity at least three times per week.[67–69]

SUMMARY

In older adults, regular exercise provides numerous health benefits that include improvements in blood pressure, diabetes, lipid profile, OA, osteoporosis, mood, neurocognitive function, and overall morbidity and mortality. Most elderly Americans do not gain this benefit because they adopt a sedentary lifestyle, often as a result of preexisting health conditions, inadequate physician education and motivation, and actual and perceived barriers to exercise.

An exercise prescription consists of aerobic exercise, strength training, balance, and flexibility training. Because the number of physician visits increases with age, it is the task of primary care providers to motivate older patients during each visit and advise them regarding regular exercise and dietary modifications. The prescription pad is a powerful tool to motivate patients on the exact frequency, duration, mode, and intensity with which to exercise. A prescription is modified depending on a patient's comorbid conditions. Motivating patients to begin exercise is best achieved by focusing on individual patient goals, concerns, and barriers to exercise. To increase compliance, discussions at each doctor's visit should ensue, and an individualized prescription outlining the patient's short- and long-term goals should be discussed.

REFERENCES

1. Malina RM. Growth, exercise, fitness and later outcomes. In: Bouchard C, Shephard RJ, Stephens T, et al, editors. Exercise, fitness and health: a consensus of current knowledge. Champaign (IL): Human Kinetics Publishers; 1990. p. 637–53.
2. Gudat U, Berger M, Lefébvre PJ. Physical activity, fitness, and non-insulin-dependent (type II) diabetes mellitus. In: Bouchard C, Shephard RJ, Stephens T, editors. Physical activity, fitness and health: International Proceedings and Consensus Statement. Champaign (IL): Human Kinetics Publishers; 1994. p. 669–83.
3. Moore S. Physical activity, fitness, and atherosclerosis. In: Bouchard C, Shephard RJ, Stephens T, editors. Physical activity, fitness, and health: International Proceedings and Consensus Statement. Champaign (IL): Human Kinetics Publishers; 1994. p. 570–8.

4. US Department of Health and Human Services. Physical activity and health. A Report of the Surgeon General. Atlanta (GA): U.S. Department of Health and Human Services, Centers for Disease Control and Prevention, National Center for Chronic Disease Prevention and Health Promotion; 1996. Available at: www.cdc.gov/nccdphp/sgr/pdf/chap5.pdf. Accessed November 12, 2003.

5. Dishman RK. Compliance/adherence in health-related exercise. Health Psychology 1982;3:237–67.

6. Singh MA. Exercise and Aging. Clin Geriatr Med 2004;20:201–21.

7. Harris BA. The influence of endurance and resistance exercise on muscle capillarization in the elderly: a review. Acta Physiol Scand 2005;185:89–97.

8. Narici MV, Reeves ND, Morse CI, et al. Muscular adaptations to resistance exercise in the elderly. Musculoskelet Neuronal Interact 2004;4:161–4.

9. Simons-Morton DG. Dose-response relationship of physical activity and cardiovascular disease risk. J Am Geriatr Soc 1998;46(2):238–40.

10. Fentem PH. Benefits of exercise in health and disease. BMJ 1994;308:1291–5.

11. Lindström J, Ilanne-Parikka P, Peltonen M, et al. Sustained reduction in the incidence of type 2 diabetes by lifestyle intervention: follow-up of the Finnish Diabetes Prevention Study. Lancet 2006;368:1673–9.

12. Church TS, Blair SN, Cocreham S, et al. Effects of aerobic and resistance training on hemoglobin A1c levels in patients with type 2 diabetes: a randomized controlled trial. JAMA 2010;304:2253–62.

13. Ettinger WH Jr, Burns R, Messier SP, et al. A randomized trial comparing aerobic exercise and resistance exercise with a health education program in older adults with knee osteoarthritis. The Fitness Arthritis and Seniors Trial (FAST). JAMA 1997;277:25–31.

14. Blumenthal JA, Babyak MA, Moore KA, et al. Effects of exercise training on older patients with major depression. Arch Intern Med 1999;159:2349–56.

15. Youngstedt SD. Effects of Exercise on Sleep. Clin Sports Med 2005;24:355–65.

16. Friedenreich CM, Cust AE. Physical activity and breast cancer risk: impact of timing, type and dose of activity and population subgroup effects. Br J Sports Med 2008;42:636–47.

17. Trojian TH, Mody K, Chain P. Exercise and colon cancer: primary and secondary prevention. Curr Sports Med Rep 2007;6:120–4.

18. Samad AK, Taylor RS, Marshall T, et al. A meta-analysis of the association of physical activity with reduced risk of colorectal cancer. Colorectal Dis 2005;7:204–13.

19. Paffenbarger RS Jr, Hyde RT, Wing AL, et al. Physical activity, all-cause mortality, and longevity of college alumni. N Engl J Med 1986;314:605–13.

20. Lee IM, Hsieh CC, Paffenbarger RS Jr. Exercise intensity and longevity in men. The Harvard Alumni Health Study. JAMA 1995;273:1179–84.

21. Huffman DM. Exercise as a calorie restriction mimetic: implications for improving healthy aging and longevity. Interdiscip Top Gerontol 2010;37:157–74.

22. Blair SN. Physical inactivity: the biggest public health problem of the 21st century. Br J Sports Med 2009;43:1, 2.

23. Cohen-Mansfield J, Marx MS, Guralnik JM. Motivators and barriers to exercise in an older community-dwelling population. J Aging Phys Act 2003;11:242–53.

24. Schutzer KA, Graves BS. Barriers and motivations to exercise in older adults. Prev Med 2004;39:1056–61.

25. Chiang K, Seman L, Belza B, et al. "It is our exercise family": experiences of ethnic older adults in a group-based exercise program. Prev Chronic Dis 2008;5:A05.

26. Cherry DK, Burt CW, Woodwell DA. National ambulatory medical care survey: 1999 summary. Advance data from vital and health statistics. No. 322. Hyattsville (MD): National Center for Health Statistics, July 2001. DHHS publication no. PHS 2001-1250 01-0383.

27. Petrella RJ, Koval JJ, Cunningham DA, et al. Can primary care doctors prescribe exercise to improve fitness? The Step Test Exercise Prescription (STEP) project. Am J Prev Med 2003;24:316–22.

28. Hornbrook MC, Stevens VJ, Wingfield DJ, et al. Preventing falls among community-dwelling older persons: results from a randomized trial. Gerontologist 1994;34:16–23.

29. Vellas BJ, Wayne SJ, Romero LJ, et al. Fear of falling and restriction of mobility in elderly fallers. Age Ageing 1997;26:189–93.

30. Fuller GF. Falls in the elderly. Am Fam Physician 2000;61:2159–68, 2173, 2174.

31. Vellas BJ, Wayne SJ, Romero L, et al. One-leg balance is an important predictor of injurious falls in older persons. J Am Geriatr Soc 1997;45:735–8.

32. Podsiadlo D, Richardson S. The timed "Up & Go": a test of basic functional mobility for frail elderly persons. J Am Geriatr Soc 1991;39:142–8.

33. Judge JO, Lindsey C, Underwood M, et al. Balance improvements in oder women: effects of exercise training. Phys Ther 1993;73:254–62 [discussion: 263–5].

34. Balducci S, Zanuso S, Nicolucci A, et al. Effect of an intensive exercise intervention strategy on modifiable cardiovascular risk factors in subjects with type 2 diabetes mellitus: a randomized controlled trial: the Italian Diabetes and Exercise Study (IDES). Arch Intern Med 2010;170:1794–803.

35. Long BJ, Calfas KJ, Wooten W, et al. A multisite field test of the acceptability of physical activity counseling in primary care: project PACE. Am J Prev Med 1996;12:73–81.

36. Mullen PD, Tabak GR. Patterns of counseling techniques used by family practice physicians for smoking, weight, exercise, and stress. Med Care 1989;27:694–704.

37. Swinburn BA, Walter LG, Arroll B, et al. The green prescription study: a randomized controlled trial of written exercise advice provided by general practitioners. Am J Public Health 1998;88:288–91.

38. Petrella RJ, Lattanzio CN, Shapiro S, et al. Improving aerobic fitness in older adults: effects of a physician-based exercise counseling and prescription program. Can Fam Physician 2010;56:e191–200.

39. Hinrichs T, Bucchi C, Brach M, et al. Feasibility of a multidimensional home-based exercise programme for the elderly with structured support given by the general practitioner's surgery: study protocol of a single arm trial preparing an RCT [ISRCTN58562962]. BMC Geriatr 2009;9:37.

40. Ingrid B, Marsella A. Factors influencing exercise participation by clients in long-term care. Perspectives 2008–2009;32(4):5–11.

41. Cooper TV, Resor MR, Stoever CJ, et al. Physical activity and physical activity adherence in the elderly based on smoking status. Addict Behav 2007;32:2268–73.

42. Calfas KJ, Long BJ, Sallis JF, et al. A controlled trial of physician counseling to promote the adoption of physical activity. Prev Med 1996;25:225–33.

43. Long BJ, Calfas KJ, Wooten W, et al. A multisite field test of the acceptability of physical activity counseling in primary care: project PACE. Am J Prev Med 1996;12:73–81.

44. Harland J, White M, Drinkwater C, et al. The Newcastle exercise project: a randomized controlled trial of methods to promote physical activity in primary care. BMJ 1999;319:828–32.

45. Lin JS, O'Connor E, Whitlock EP, et al. Behavioral counseling to promote physical activity and a healthful diet to prevent cardiovascular disease in adults: a systematic review for the U.S. Preventive Services Task Force. Ann Intern Med 2010;153:736–50.

46. King AC, Friedman R, Marcus B, et al. Ongoing physical activity advice by humans versus computers: the Community Health Advice by Telephone (CHAT) trial. Health Psychol 2007;26:718–27.
47. Kerse NM, Flicker L, Jolley D, et al. Improving the health behaviours of elderly people: randomized controlled trial of a general practice education programme. BMJ 1999; 319:683–7.
48. Phillips EM, Schneider JC, Mercer GR. Motivating elders to initiate exercise. Arch Phys Med Rehabil 2004;85(Suppl 3):S52–7.
49. Litt MD, Kleppinger A, Judge JO. Initiation and maintenance of exercise behavior in the older women: predictors from the social learning model. J Behav Med 2002;25: 83–97.
50. American College of Sports Medicine. AHA/ACSM Joint Position Statement: Recommendations for Cardiovascular Screening, Staffing, and Emergency Policies at Health/Fitness Facilities. In: Balady GJ, Chairman B, Driscoll D, et al, editors. ACSM's Health/Fitness Facility Standards and Guidelines. 3rd edition. Champaign (IL): Human Kinetics Publishers; 2006. Appendix G, p. 173.
51. Haskell WL, Lee IM, Pate RR, et al. Physical activity and public health: updated recommendation for adults from the American College of Sports Medicine and the American Heart Association. Med Sci Sports Exerc 2007;39:1423–34.
52. American College of Sports Medicine. ACSM's guidelines for exercise testing and prescription. 6th edition. Philadelphia: Lippincott Williams & Wilkins; 2000. p. 156–8.
53. Larson EB, Wang L, Bowen JD, et al. Exercise is associated with reduced risk for incident dementia among persons 65 years of age and older. Ann Intern Med 2006;144:73–81.
54. Yaffe K, Barnes D, Nevitt M, et al. A prospective study of physical activity and cognitive decline in elderly women: women who walk. Arch Intern Med 2001;161:1703–8.
55. Weuve J, Kang JH, Manson JE, et al. Physical activity, including walking, and cognitive function in older women. JAMA 2004;292:1454–61.
56. Abbott RD, White LR, Ross GW, et al. Walking and dementia in physically capable elderly men. JAMA 2004;292:1447–53.
57. Heyn P, Abreu BC, Ottenbacher KJ. The effects of exercise training on elderly persons with cognitive impairment and dementia: a meta-analysis. Arch Phys Med Rehabil 2004;85:1694–704.
58. Buettner LL, Lundegren H, Lago D, et al. Therapeutic recreation as an intervention for persons with dementia and agitation: An efficacy study. Am J Alzheimers Dis Other 1996;11:4–12.
59. Slemenda C, Brandt KD, Heilman DK, et al. Quadriceps weakness and osteoarthritis of the knee. Ann Intern Med 1997;127:97–104.
60. Slemenda C, Heilman DK, Brandt KD, et al. Reduced quadriceps strength relative to body weight: a risk factor for knee osteoarthritis in women? Arthritis Rheum 1998;41: 1951–9.
61. American Thoracic Society. ATS Documents: Statements, Guidelines & Reports. Standards for the Diagnosis and Care of Patients with Chronic Obstructive Pulmonary Disease; 1995. Available at http://www.thoracic.org/statements/resources/archive/ standards-for-the-diagnosis-and-care-of-patients-with-chronic-obstructive-pulmonary-disease-1995.pdf. Accessed march 10, 2011.
62. Cooper CB. Exercise in chronic pulmonary disease: aerobic exercise prescription. Med Sci Sports Exerc 2001; 33(7 Suppl):S671–9.
63. Puhan M, Scharplatz M, Troosters T, et al. Pulmonary rehabilitation following exacerbations of chronic obstructive pulmonary disease. Cochrane Database Syst Rev 2009;1:CD005305.

64. Fleg JL. Exercise therapy for elderly heart failure patients. Clin Geriatr Med 2007;23: 221–34.
65. Lloyd-Jones D, Adams RJ, Brown TM, et al. Heart disease and stroke statistics— 2010 update: a report from the American Heart Association. Circulation 2010;121: e46–e215.
66. Vasan RS, Larson MG, Leip EP, et al. Impact of high-normal blood pressure on the risk of cardiovascular disease. N Engl J Med 2001;345:1291–7.
67. Gribbin B, Pickering TG, Sleight P, et al. Effect of age and high blood pressure on baroreflex sensitivity in man. Circ Res 1971;29:424–31.
68. Madden KM, Lockhart C, Cuff D, et al. Short-term aerobic exercise reduces arterial stiffness in older adults with type 2 diabetes, hypertension, and hypercholesterolemia. Diabetes Care 2009;32:1531–5.
69. Westhoff TH, Franke N, Schmidt S, et al. Too old to benefit from sports? The cardiovascular effects of exercise training in elderly subjects treated for isolated systolic hypertension. Blood Press Res 2007;30:240–7.

Fatigue and Chronic Fatigue in the Elderly: Definitions, Diagnoses, and Treatments

Vincent Morelli, MD

KEYWORDS

- Elderly • Fatigue • Chronic • Diagnosis • Treatment

Because fatigue is so prevalent in the elderly (>70%),[1] it is included as a specific topic in this publication on successful aging. It is presented so that the primary care physician may help optimize elderly patients' lives, to maximize their level of function and engagement with life.

Fatigue may be generally categorized as recent (<1 month), prolonged (1–6 months), or chronic (>6 months).[2] It is perceived by patients to be either (1) inability to initiate activity—a perception of generalized weakness in the absence of objective findings; (2) a reduced capacity to maintain activity—easy fatigability; or (3) difficulty with concentration, memory, and emotional stability (mental fatigue).[3]

A 2010 review[1] proposed that fatigue may be predominantly mental (cognitive or emotional) or physical (sleepiness, lack of energy, and weakness), or both. The authors of this study and of several others[4–12] propose that "quality of fatigue" scales are also useful in work-up, treatment, and patient follow-up.

Because fatigue (recent, prolonged, or chronic) has been reported in up to 20% of primary care visits,[13–17] it is important that the physician be well versed in the evaluation and management of this complaint.

In primary care, the diagnosis of most patients with fatigue will fall into the categories of recent or prolonged fatigue, whereas only a minority will have symptoms that progress beyond 6 months. Further, these "chronic" patients may be categorized with either chronic fatigue syndrome (CFS) as defined by the Centers for Disease Control and Prevention (CDC; see later), or with idiopathic fatigue (IF) if symptoms have been present for more than 6 months but do not fit the strict CDC definition of CFS.

Chronic fatigue syndrome, as defined by the CDC in 1994,[18] requires that:

- Fatigue be present for at least 6 months.
- Fatigue *not* be caused by other medical conditions, substance abuse within the last 2 years, obesity (BMI > 45), or *major* psychiatric conditions.

Department of Family and Community Medicine, Meharry Medical College, 1005 Dr D.B. Todd, Jr, Boulevard, Nashville, TN 37208, USA
E-mail address: vmorelli@mmc.edu

Clin Geriatr Med 27 (2011) 673–686
doi:10.1016/j.cger.2011.07.011
0749-0690/11/$ – see front matter © 2011 Elsevier Inc. All rights reserved.

geriatric.theclinics.com

In addition to these two requirements, four or more of the following eight findings *must* be present:

1. Postexertional malaise
2. Impaired memory or concentration
3. Sore throat
4. Tender glands
5. Aching or stiff muscles
6. Joint pain
7. Headaches
8. Unrefreshing sleep.

If symptoms have persisted for more than 6 months but at least four of these eight findings are not present, the patient is categorized as having idiopathic fatigue.

Several major psychiatric disorders preclude a diagnosis of CFS, including psychosis, major depression, bipolar disorder, schizophrenia, dementia, delusional disorders, and eating disorders. Fatigue in these conditions may be attributed to the underlying psychoemotional conditions instead of CFS. Of note, a diagnosis of "common" depression or dysthymia is not excluded; therefore, CFS and "common depression" may coexist. A 2009 survey of 1045 CFS patients found 36% had concomitant depression,[19] and other studies are confirmatory, noting that roughly one-third to one-half of CFS patients will have concomitant depression.[20,21] This may be why so many primary care physicians attribute CFS and IF to psychological causes and why roughly only half of primary care physicians believe CFS exists.[22] In theory, however, if "common depression" patients with CFS were adequately treated for depression, their mood would elevate but their CFS would remain.

DEMOGRAPHICS AND WHY THIS ARTICLE IS INCLUDED IN A PUBLICATION ON SUCCESSFUL AGING

Although the exact total prevalence of all forms of fatigue (recent, prolonged, or chronic) is unknown owing to underreporting,[23] estimates of *chronic fatigue* range from 0.006% to 3.0% in the general population,[13,24–26] indicating that more than a million people may be affected by chronic fatigue in the United States alone.[27]

Although young (aged 30–40), white, successful women may complain of isolated fatigue more frequently than persons in other demographic groups, this seems to be due to increased access to care rather that an actual higher prevalence within this group. In fact, several community surveys have found that Latinos, African Americans, other minorities, and those in lower educational or socioeconomic strata have significantly higher prevalence rates than whites.[27,28] The authors of these surveys suggest that the increased prevalence of fatigue in these cohorts may be due to poorer general health or the increased "general life stress" experienced on the lower rungs of the educational/socioeconomic ladder.

Most surveys and studies find a significantly higher prevalence of CFS in women (some as high as 75%) and record the mean duration of the disease as 3 to 9 years.[27–30] Physician attitudes regarding fatigue and CFS vary, but in 2000 Steven and colleagues[31] demonstrated that one-third of 2000 general practitioners surveyed did not believe that CFS was a distinct syndrome and thought the most likely cause was depression.

Another recent survey of 811 primary care physicians in Britain revealed that 41% did not feel confident in CFS treatment, and only 12% enjoyed working with CFS patients.[32]

As stated previously, surveys of primary care practices indicate that 10% to 20% of primary care patients complain of fatigue (not necessarily chronic fatigue)[13,33] and, of those seeking medical attention, roughly two-thirds may be expected to have a medical or psychiatric cause for fatigue.[13] The remaining one-third will have no identifiable cause.

In the aging population, the complaint of fatigue is often overlooked by caregivers because of other more pressing medical needs. However, it is important to recognize that when specifically questioned, 70% of older primary care patients (average age 74 years) report fatigue, and 43% report feeling tired most of the time.[1] In addition to being an isolated complaint in this population, fatigue is also (obviously) associated with chronic medical conditions including heart disease, pulmonary disease, neurologic maladies, musculoskeletal conditions, diabetes and endocrine disorders, rheumatologic conditions, infectious diseases, cancer, immune disorders, and as a side effect of medications. Medical conditions contributing to fatigue are discussed in the sections that follow.

NORMAL FATIGUE WITH AGING

Generally with normal aging, the response and recovery times are slower for all of the organ systems. This is not fatigue per se but instead is referred to as "lower reserve capacity." Normal effects of aging include changes in several parameters at the cellular level and several contributory factors at the organ system level including:

- Nervous system: increased reaction time and reduced CNS receptors
- Cardiovascular system: increase in blood pressure and a decrease in maximal achievable heart rate, cardiac output, and $\dot{V}o_2$max
- Respiratory system: decreased vital capacity, lung compliance, and thoracic mobility
- Musculoskeletal system: decreased bone mass, lean body mass, and fast twitch (type 2) muscle fibers and increased stiffness of tendons and cartilage.

Although all of these changes may be expected to increase fatigability in the elderly, there is no agreement on what constitutes "normal fatigue" and obviously vast individual differences can and do occur.

CHRONIC FATIGUE SYNDROME

To meet the strict definition of CFS, patients must meet the CDC criteria. As mentioned previously, there is little difference in the primary care physician's approach to fatigue that is recent, prolonged, chronic, or idiopathic. For the primary care physician the evaluation of fatigue is usually the same regardless of how much time has elapsed since the onset of symptoms, although treatment will vary with diagnostic categorization.

Clinical Manifestations

Patients ultimately diagnosed with CFS present initially with severe fatigue and an average of eight additional complaints.[34] The complaints range from those included in the CDC definition (eg, impaired memory, difficulty concentrating, headaches, joint pains, myalgias) to more nonspecific symptoms including dizziness, nausea, gastrointestinal problems, and night sweats.

Many patients presenting to tertiary care centers tell of an acute onset of symptoms following an infectious malady[35,36]; however, most reporting to primary care centers note a gradual onset of symptoms.[37]

Attempts To Identify An Etiology

Although several CFS-like cases were described in the 1800s and early 1900s,[38] interest in the syndrome rose dramatically in the 1980s when a possible association with neurologic or infectious etiologies seemed plausible. Etiologies explored during recent years have been viral causative agents, neurologic dysfunction, endocrine imbalances,[39] immune causes, sleep disorders, genetic causes, circadian rhythm disturbances,[40–42] and psychological predispositions. Despite careful investigations, no clear common pathogenesis has been identified. Authorities now generally believe the cause of CFS to be multifactorial, possibly representing an end outward manifestation elicited by several contributing factors or disease processes.[43]

A Primary Care Approach To CFS

Despite its unclear etiology, primary care physicians may be helped in their approach to CFS patients by examining factors that: (a) predispose to the syndrome; (b) precipitate the syndrome; or (c) perpetuate the syndrome. This approach was set out by Lancet in a 2006 review,[30] and although it is often difficult to know if a factor (eg, depressive personality type) predisposes, precipitates, or perpetuates CFS, categorization in this manner still may be helpful to the practicing clinician.

Predisposing Factors

Predisposing factors for CFS may include personality abnormalities such as introverted personality, higher levels of worry,[44] increased harm avoidance, decreased self-directedness, poor levels of cooperativeness, high degree of perfectionism, depressive personality, and neuroticism[45,46] (a tendency to experience negative emotional states such as anxiety, anger, guilt, and depression longer and more intensely). Individuals who respond poorly to stress, have poor emotional regulation, or exhibit poor interpersonal skills may also be predisposed to CFS.

Although personality disorders are not present in all CFS patients, Henderson and Tannock,[47] Ciccone and colleagues,[21] and Johnson and colleagues[48] found a high level of these maladies (39% in CFS compared to 10% in the general population) in their subjects. The predominant types found were obsessive–compulsive, histrionic, and borderline personality disorders.

The high levels of these predisposing factors, though not causative, highlight the idea that all CFS patients might be helped by a careful psychological evaluation.

Precipitating Factors

A recent survey[36] examined the events that may have precipitated the onset of CFS in 134 patients. The researchers found that 72% of patients believed that they had experienced some sort of infection before the onset of symptoms. Infections that have been implicated, among others, include infectious mononucleosis, Lyme disease, Q fever,[49] brucellosis, hepatitis, cat-scratch, genital herpes, and zoster.[36]

In the aforementioned survey,[36] of the 28% of patients who recalled no inciting infection, 40% thought that other precipitating factors such as trauma, allergies, or surgery had induced their fatigue, whereas 60% could not elucidate any inciting events.

In other studies, the onset of CFS has been associated with psychological stressors.[50,51]

Perpetuating Factors

Several factors may impede recovery in CFS patients. Attributing the cause to a physical factor,[52] inactivity, avoidance of activities that provoke symptoms, a poor sense of control,[53] lack of social support, or overly solicitous responses from significant others[54] may all contribute to prolonged fatigue.

In addition, the physician–patient relationship may also perpetuate symptoms if physicians encourage excessive medical testing or, conversely, if they continue to attribute CFS to psychological causes.[55] It seems the primary care physician must walk a fine line with little precise guidance.

All of the preceding patient and physician factors must be taken into consideration if the primary care physician is to manage these patients optimally.

Disease Course and Prognosis

A recent review noted that full recovery in CFS patients is unlikely.[29] A median of 7% of patients can expect full recovery with treatment; only 39% of patients can expect improvement in symptoms in the medium term (12–40 months). However, the likelihood of improvement and full recovery increases with increased study period. One survey showed that 48% of patients displayed complete recovery at a 10-year follow-up.[56]

However, the above bleak prognosis may not reflect CFS seen in the primary care setting, where symptoms are generally less chronic and less severe. In this setting, one study found a 20% recovery and a 60% improvement rate during a 1- to 7-year follow up.[57]

Substantiating this 60% improvement rate, an early longitudinal study of unexplained fatigue (fatigue present for at least 6 weeks; study conducted before the 1994 CDC definition of CFS) showed that two-thirds of patients improve spontaneously in the first 2 years but that those whose illness duration is greater than 2 years tend to stay unwell.[58] These studies may better reflect the expected prognosis of patients seen in primary care centers.

Treatment

Before discussing treatment of CFS patients, it should be noted that patients are generally *not* satisfied with the care for their condition. A 2001 survey found that two-thirds of patients with CFS were dissatisfied with the quality of medical care. Patients stated that confusion over diagnosis; relegation of their illness to a psychological category; and dismissive, skeptical, or inadequately educated physicians were the main reasons for their dissatisfaction. Authors of the study urged better physician–patient communication, more skillful use of interpersonal skills, and improved physician education as a means to improve patient satisfaction and treatment outcomes.[59] Three more recent surveys (2005, 2005, 2009) substantiated these findings and noted that only 23% to 41% of primary care physicians thought they had sufficient knowledge of CFS. All authors note that CFS is not adequately addressed by the medical community.[32,60,61]

General treatment goals include helping patients to:

- Accomplish activities of daily living
- Return to work
- Maintain interpersonal relationships
- Perform daily exercise.

Brief, regularly scheduled appointments are generally recommended, though no studies have addressed optimal frequency of follow-up.

Several treatments have been tried in CFS, including cognitive–behavioral therapy, graded exercise therapy, immunologic treatment, hydrocortisone, pharmacologic therapy, supplements, and complementary/alternative treatments. Some of these are discussed in the text that follows. In addition, it must be remembered that because CFS might represent the end result of several different disease processes, treatment methods may not be effective in all patients. In future clinical trials, patient selection and categorization will be paramount in treatment selection.

Cognitive–behavioral therapy

Two recent studies, in 2008 and 2010,[62,63] revealed that roughly 38% of patients with CFS were significantly helped by cognitive–behavioral therapy (CBT), at a cost of approximately $6700 per recovered patient. These authors considered the cost acceptable and endorsed CBT.

A 2008 Cochrane database review[64] concluded that CBT was significantly better than "usual" intervention, with 40% of CFS patients helped by CBT whereas only 26% of those under usual care improved. However, it was noted that data collected at follow-up after the conclusion of CBT treatment were insufficient to validate the use of CBT over the longer term. Contrary to earlier studies and reviews, the most recent review of CBT (2009)[65] concluded that CBT was ineffective in CFS.

In summary, we must conclude that, at best, a modest improvement with CBT can be expected in CFS patients.

Graded exercise therapy

The latest randomized trial of 61 patients showed graded exercise therapy (GET) superior to stretching/relaxation in the treatment of CFS.[66] Several other studies have substantiated the beneficial effects of GET in CFS at up to 2-year follow-up.[67,68] The most recent Cochrane review on GET (2004) noted that, "There is encouraging evidence that some patients may benefit from exercise therapy and no evidence that exercise therapy may worsen outcomes on average." However, they found that patients tended to drop out of exercise programs frequently.[26]

Diet

Although the lay literature has claimed that a high-yeast diet may cause or exacerbate CFS, no rigorous study has validated this claim. The one well conducted randomized trial in this arena failed to demonstrate any benefit from a low-sugar–low-yeast diet[69] over a 6-month study period in 51 patients with CFS.[70]

Nor has any benefit been demonstrated for spirulina, an algae supplement commonly touted for its curative effects in CFS.[71]

Of interest and possibly an area for further study, one trial recently noted that 19 of 30 patients with fibromyalgia (often said to be closely related to CFS) significantly improved on a vegetarian diet.[72]

In summary, to date, no studies have substantiated that any specific dietary measure improves outcome in patients with CFS. Also, interestingly, in our research on diet and CFS, we were surprised that we could find no surveys or studies that carefully examined dietary practices in fatigue or CFS patients.

Antidepressants

Citalopram (Lexapro) has shown possible use in CFS patients in two small (N = 16 and N = 32) trials[73,74] Patients in these trials exhibited improvement in fatigue and in depression scores, but the studies were suboptimal and the latest was a nonrandomized open-label study.

The only well performed study we could find examining the use of antidepressants in CFS was conducted In 1996 and published in Lancet.[75] In this double-blinded study, CFS patients were randomized to receive either 20 mg of fluoxetine (Prozac) per day or placebo. No differences were found over the 8-week trial period. We could find no other significant studies that substantiated a significant benefit of antidepressants in CFS.

Supplements

Melatonin. Because melatonin secretion has been noted to be delayed in some CFS patients, a recent open-label study[76] was performed to assess the effect of supplemental melatonin on 29 CFS patients. The researchers noted a significant improvement of fatigue symptoms in patients treated with melatonin supplementation (5 mg) 5 to 8 hours before bedtime, but no randomized trials substantiating this claim have been conducted.

Magnesium. These supplements were found to have an overall beneficial effect in one good-quality randomized controlled trial.[77] Patients with CFS had been noted to have low erythrocyte magnesium levels (red cell magnesium is more indicative of intercellular magnesium levels than serum levels because serum levels are maintained at the expense of intracellular stores); thus, 32 patients were randomized to receive either IM magnesium sulfate (1 g every week) or placebo for 6 weeks. Twelve of 15 patients in the treatment group noted improvement whereas only 3 of the 17 placebo group did. Magnesium deficiency is known to cause neuro/psychological symptoms, and it is known that physical inactivity, stress, anxiety, and nervousness can lead to hypomagnesemia. However, the basis for the therapeutic action of magnesium in CFS is unknown.

Fatty acids. This type of supplementation has been shown to improve joint pain, morning stiffness, and fatigue in patients with rheumatoid arthritis[78]; thus, it seems reasonable to consider such supplementation in CFS patients as well.

As further rationale to this line of thinking, because omega-6 polyunsaturated fatty acids (PUFAs) have been found to be increased in CFS, one study suggested that increased omega-6 PUFAs and decreased omega-3 PUFAs could play a role in the pathophysiology of CFS, forming the rationale for omega-3 supplementation. In addition, researchers found that the omega-3/omega-6 ratio significantly and negatively correlates to the severity of CFS, again suggesting that a decreased availability of omega-3 PUFAs could play a role in the pathophysiology of CFS, and that patients with CFS could respond favorably to treatment with omega-3 PUFAs.[79]

Despite early studies demonstrating theoretical promise for fatty acid supplementation in patients with post viral fatigue,[80,81] later studies failed to show any consistent benefit from fatty acid supplementation.[82]

Amino acids. The essential amino acid L-ornithine is a breakdown product of arginine, part of the urea cycle which is necessary for the disposal of excess nitrogen and ammonia formed during exercise.[83,84] L-ornithine has been shown to improve both objective and subjective measures of fatigue caused by exercise.[85] Despite this, however, no use of amino acid supplementation in CFS has been noted in the literature.

L-Carnitine. L-Carnitine is used in the transport of fatty acids into the mitochondria for energy production and has been reported to be decreased in CFS patients.[86] With this in mind, studies have been undertaken to see what efficacy L-carnitine supplementation might have in CFS. In one study of 30 patients, L-carnitine was found to be beneficial in CFS patients. Another small study (N = 36) reported improvement in multiple sclerosis patients with fatigue when supplemented with L-carnitine (1 g twice a day).[87] In a final randomized blinded study done in 2008,[88] 96 subjects aged 70 years and older, with persistent fatigue, were given either L-carnitine supplementation (2 g twice a day) or placebo for 6 months. Results demonstrated a significant improvement in both physical and mental fatigue and sleep disturbances in patients supplemented with L-carnitine. These studies are small, and it is difficult to make generalizations, but L-carnitine appears to be beneficial and safe.

Immunotherapy

Contrary to early studies validating the usefulness of intravenous immunoglobulin (IVIG) in CFS patients,[89] later definitive studies found no benefit from three different doses of IVIG, given monthly over a 3-month trial period.[90]

α-Interferon. In a 1996 double-blinded crossover trial of 26 patients with CFS, α-interferon was found to have no benefit over placebo.[91] We could find no subsequent studies demonstrating any benefit.

Corticosteroids

An early study,[92] using relatively high doses of cortisone (25–35 mg/day, dosed 20–30 mg every morning, and 5 mg by mouth every evening) found a mild improvement of symptoms in CFS patients when steroids were taken over a 12-week study period. However, evidence of adrenal suppression occurred in a high percentage of treatment arm patients, and authors felt that the potential adverse effects of steroids may outweigh any benefits.

A subsequent 1999 double-blind crossover trial of 32 CFS patients without comorbid psychiatric conditions randomized patients to receive either *low-dose cortisol* (5–10 mg cortisone every morning; the equivalent of 1–2.5 mg of prednisone) or placebo for a month. Results noted reduced fatigue scores in those taking prednisone. In this study, 28% of the cortisone treatment arm returned to normal levels of fatigue and no difference in response was observed between the different doses (5 or 10 mg). In addition, the use of *low doses* did not cause a significant suppression of endogenous cortisol.[93]

Finally, the latest randomized crossover study, conducted in 2003, treated 80 CFS patients (as previously, screened to rule out comorbid psychiatric conditions) for a total of 6 months, but revealed no improvement of fatigue from that obtained using low-dose steroids (5 mg of hydrodcortisone per day plus 50 μg daily of 9-alfa-fludrocortisone).[94]

In comparing the latest two trials, it should be noted that patients in the final study (the one reporting no improvement with steroids) had a rather long duration of fatigue (average of 30 months; most studies have shown that the longer the fatigue is present the more resistant to treatment) and that the duration of fatigue was not reported in the former study (the one reporting improvement with steroids). Also, in the former study, an inclusion criterion was that the fatigue must have commenced over a brief, 6-week period. These facts, taken together, may indicate that fatigue of short duration or acute onset (fatigue also more likely to improve on its own) may be helped by steroids while that of longer duration or gradual onset may be more resistant to treatment.

No clinical trials with low-dose steroids have been performed after 2003, and we could find no studies examining the use of short-course, high-dose steroids.

Stimulants

In a recent study,[95] methylphenidate (Ritalin, Concerta), 10 mg twice a day, was given to 60 CFS patients with fatigue and concentration difficulties. The 4-week randomized crossover noted that fatigue and concentration measures improved significantly in the treatment arm as compared to placebo. A clinically significant improvement (>33%) was noted in 17% of patients in terms of fatigue, and 22% of patients were significantly helped in terms of concentration. The authors noted (again) that those whose fatigue was less chronic responded better. They also noted that more studies are needed to investigate the long-term effects and side effects of this treatment.

In another trial, dexamphetamine (essentially Adderall) was given to 20 CFS patients in a short (6 weeks) randomized trial. Improvements in fatigue were noted in nine of ten treatment arm patients and only four of ten patients in the placebo group. The authors recommended further large-scale trials to gauge true efficacy.[96]

Modafinil (Provigil) was also tried in a single trial and was not shown to benefit CFS patients with either physical or mental fatigue when given at doses of 200 to 400 mg every day.[97]

SUMMARY

A specific cause for fatigue in two-thirds of primary care patients can be found after a careful history and physical and laboratory examination. Treatment in such cases should be directed toward the underlying cause or contributing conditions. When fatigue is classified as either chronic or idiopathic, proper treatment is less clear. Because CFS is thought to be the end manifestation of several different maladies, no single treatment plan is optimal for all patients. First, a psychiatric evaluation on all patients with chronic or idiopathic fatigue should be performed. Because 40% of CFS patients have a concomitant predisposing personality disorder, and 33% to 50% have concomitant depression, this seems warranted. In addition, some nonpharmacologic measures to consider in selected patients include cognitive behavioral therapy, graded exercise therapy, vitamin B_{12}, magnesium, melatonin, L-carnitine, elimination diets, vegetarian diets, and vitamin D. Pharmaceutical options to include stimulants such as Ritalin, Concerta or Addreall, antidepressants such as Lexapro (not Prozac), and low-dose steroids (2.5 of prednisone every day). As with any treatment, but especially the treatment of "syndromes," which by definition are of unclear etiology, the side effects and risk/benefit ratios must be considered.

REFERENCES

1. Hardy SE. Qualities of fatigue and associated chronic conditions among older adults. J Pain Symptom Manage 2010;39:1033–42.
2. Sánchez Rodríguez A, González Maroño C, Sánchez Ledesma M. Chronic fatigue syndrome: a syndrome in search of definition. Rev Clin Esp 2005;205:70–74.
3. Markowitz AJ, Rabow MW. Palliative management of fatigue at the close of life: "it feels like my body is just worn out." JAMA 2007;298:217.
4. Poluri A, Mores J, Cook DB, et al. Fatigue in the elderly population. Phys Med Rehabil Clin N Am 2005;16:91–108.
5. Okuyama T, Akechi T, Kugaya A, et al. Development and validation of the cancer fatigue scale: a brief, three-dimensional, self-rating scale for assessment of fatigue in cancer patients. J Pain Symptom Manage 2000;19:5–14.
6. Piper BF, Dibble SL, Dodd MJ, et al. The revised Piper Fatigue Scale: psychometric evaluation in women with breast cancer. Oncol Nurs Forum 1998;25:677–84.

7. Smets EM, Garssen B, Bonke B, et al. The multidimensional Fatigue Inventory (MFI) psychometric qualities of an instrument to assess fatigue. J Psychosom Res 1995; 39:315–25.

8. Stein KD, Martin SC, Hann DM, et al. A multidimensional measure of fatigue for use with cancer patients. Cancer Pract 1998;6:143–52.

9. Holley SK. Evaluating patient distress from cancer-related fatigue: an instrument development study. Oncol Nurs Forum 2000;27:1425–31.

10. Fisk JD, Ritvo PG, Ross L, et al. Measuring the functional impact of fatigue: initial validation of the fatigue impact scale. Clin Infect Dis 1994;18(Suppl 1):S79–83.

11. Schwartz AL. The Schwartz Cancer Fatigue Scale: testing reliability and validity. Oncol Nurs Forum 1998;25:711–7.

12. Whitehead L. The measurement of fatigue in chronic illness: a systematic review of unidimensional and multidimensional fatigue measures. J Pain Symptom Manage 2009;37:107–28.

13. Bates DW, Schmitt W, Buchwald D, et al. Prevalence of fatigue and chronic fatigue syndrome in a primary care practice. Arch Intern Med 1993;153:2759–65.

14. Cathebras PJ, Robbins JM, Kirmayer LJ, et al. Fatigue in primary care: prevalence, psychiatric comorbidity, illness behavior, and outcome. J Gen Intern Med 1992;7: 276–86.

15. David A, Pelosi A, McDonald E, et al. Tired, weak, or in need of rest: a profile of fatigue among general practice attenders. BMJ 1990;301:1199–202.

16. Kroenke K, Wood DR, Mangelsdorff D, et al. Chronic fatigue in primary care: prevalence, patient characteristics, and outcome. JAMA 1988;260:929–34.

17. McDonald E, David AS, Pelosi AJ, et al. Chronic fatigue in primary care attenders. Psychol Med 1993;23:987–98.

18. Fukuda K, Straus SE, Hickie I, et al. The chronic fatigue syndrome: a comprehensive approach to its definition and study. International Chronic Fatigue Syndrome Study Group. Ann Intern Med 1994;121:953–9.

19. Fuller-Thomson E, Nimigon J. Factors associated with depression among individuals with chronic fatigue syndrome: findings from a nationally representative survey. Fam Pract 2008;25(6):414–22.

20. Johnson SK, DeLuca J, Natelson BH. Depression in fatiguing illness: comparing patients with chronic fatigue syndrome, multiple sclerosis and depression. J Affect Disord 1996;39:21–30.

21. Ciccone DS, Busichio K, Vickroy M, et al. Psychiatric morbidity in the chronic fatigue syndrome: are patients with personality disorder more physically impaired? J Psychosom Res 2003;54:445–52.

22. Darbishire L, Ridsdale L, Seed PT. Distinguishing patients with chronic fatigue from those with chronic fatigue syndrome: a diagnostic study in UK primary care. Br J Gen Pract 2003;53:441–5.

23. Wick JY, LaFleur J. Fatigue: implications for the elderly. Consult Pharm 2007;22:566– 70, 573–4, 576–8.

24. Wessely S, Chalder T, Hirsch S, et al. The prevalence and morbidity of chronic fatigue and the chronic fatigue syndrome: a prospective primary care study. Am J Public Health 1997;87:1449–55.

25. Reyes M, Gary HE Jr, Dobbins JG, et al. Surveillance for chronic fatigue syndrome— four US cities, September 1989 through August 1993. MMWR CDC Surveill Summ 1997;46:1–13.

26. Edmonds M, McGuire H, Price J. Exercise therapy for chronic fatigue syndrome. Cochrane Database Syst Rev 2004;3:CD003200.

27. Jason LA, Richman JA, Rademaker AW, et al. A community-based study of chronic fatigue syndrome. Arch Intern Med 1999;159:2129–37.
28. Steele L, Dobbins JG, Fukuda K, et al. The epidemiology of chronic fatigue in San Francisco. Am J Med 1998;105:83S–90S.
29. Cairns R, Hotopf M. A systematic review describing the prognosis of chronic fatigue syndrome. Occup Med (Lond) 2005;55:20–31.
30. Prins JB, van der Meer JW, Bleijenberg G. Chronic fatigue syndrome. Lancet 2006:367:346–55.
31. Steven ID, McGrath B, Qureshi F, et al. General practitioners' beliefs, attitudes and reported actions towards chronic fatigue syndrome. Aust Fam Physician 2000;29: 80–5.
32. Bowen J, Pheby D, Charlett A, et al. Chronic fatigue syndrome: a survey of GPs' attitudes and knowledge. Fam Pract 2005;22:389–93.
33. Pawlikowska T, Chalder T, Hirsch SR, et al. Population based study of fatigue and psychological distress. BMJ 1994;308:763–6.
34. Vercoulen JH, Swanink CM, Fennis JF, et al. Dimensional assessment of chronic fatigue syndrome. J Psychosom Res 1994;38:383–92.
35. Schluederberg A, Straus SE, Peterson P, et al. Chronic fatigue syndrome research: definition and medical outcome assessment. Ann Intern Med 1992;117:325–31.
36. Salit IE. Precipitating factors for the chronic fatigue syndrome, J Psychiatr Res 1997;31:59–65.
37. Solomon L, Reeves WC. Factors influencing the diagnosis of chronic fatigue syndrome. Arch Intern Med 2004;164:2241–45.
38. Shorter E. The epidemic of chronic fatigue. In: From paralysis to fatigue: a history of psychosomatic illness in the modern era. New York: Free Press; 1992. p. 307–14.
39. Cleare AJ. The neuroendocrinology of chronic fatigue syndrome. Endocr Rev 2003; 24:236–52.
40. Moldofsky H. Sleep, neuroimmune and neuroendocrine functions in fibromyalgia and chronic fatigue syndrome. Adv Neuroimmunol 1995;5:39–56.
41. Parker AJ, Wessely S, Cleare AJ. The neuroendocrinology of chronic fatigue syndrome and fibromyalgia. Psychol Med 2001;31:1331–45.
42. Racciatti D, Guagnano MT, Vecchiet J, et al. Chronic fatigue syndrome: circadian rhythm and hypothalamic-pituitary-adrenal (HPA) axis impairment. Int J Immunopathol Pharmacol 2001;14:11–15.
43. Cleare AJ. The HPA axis and the genesis of chronic fatigue syndrome. Trends Endocrinol Metabol 2004;15:55–9.
44. Taillefer SS, Kirmayer LJ, Robbins JM, et al. Correlates of illness worry in chronic fatigue syndrome. J Psychosom Res 2003;54:331–7.
45. Buckley L, MacHale SM, Cavanagh JT, et al. Personality dimensions in chronic fatigue syndrome and depression. J Psychosom Res 1999;46:395–400.
46. van Geelen SM, Sinnema G, Hermans HJ, et al. Personality and chronic fatigue syndrome: methodological and conceptual issues. Clin Psychol Rev 2007;27:885–903.
47. Henderson M, Tannock C. Objective assessment of personality disorder in chronic fatigue syndrome. J Psychosom Res 2004;56:251–4.
48. Johnson SK, DeLuca J, Natelson BH. Chronic fatigue syndrome: reviewing the research findings. Ann Behav Med 1999;21:258–71.
49. Lloyd AR. Postinfective fatigue. In: Jason LA, Fennell PA, Taylor RR, editors. Handbook of chronic fatigue syndrome. Hoboken (NJ): John Wiley & Sons; 2003. p. 108–123.

50. Hatcher S, House A. Life events, difficulties and dilemmas in the onset of chronic fatigue syndrome: a case-control study. Psychol Med 2003;33:1185–92.

51. Theorell T, Blomkvist V, Lindh G, et al. Critical life events, infections, and symptoms during the year preceding chronic fatigue syndrome (CFS): an examination of CFS patients and subjects with a nonspecific life crisis. Psychosom Med 1999;61:304–10.

52. Vercoulen JH, Swanink CM, Galama JM, et al. The persistence of fatigue in chronic fatigue syndrome and multiple sclerosis: the development of a model. J Psychosom Res 1998:45:507–17.

53. Moss-Morris R, Petrie KJ, Weinman J. Functioning in chronic fatigue syndrome: do illness perceptions play a regulatory role? Br J Health Psychol 1996;1:15–25.

54. Schmaling KD, Smith WR, Buchwald DS. Significant other responses are associated with fatigue and functional status among patients with chronic fatigue syndrome. Psychosom Med 2000;62:444–50.

55. Stanley I, Salmon P, Peters S. Doctors and social epidemics: the problem of persistent unexplained physical symptoms, including chronic fatigue. Br J Gen Pract 2002;52:355–6.

56. Reyes M, Dobbins JG, Nisenbaum R, et al. Chronic fatigue syndrome progression and self-defined recovery: evidence from the CDC surveillance system. J Chronic Fatigue Syndrome 1999;5:17–27.

57. Saltzstein BJ, Wyshak G, Hubbuch JT, et al. A naturalistic study of the chronic fatigue syndrome among women in primary care. Gen Hosp Psychiatry 1998;20:307–16.

58. Sharpe M, Hawton K, Seagroatt V, et al. Follow-up of patients presenting with fatigue to an infectious diseases clinic. BMJ 1992;305:147–52.

59. Deale A, Wessely S. Patients' perceptions of medical care in chronic fatigue syndrome. Soc Sci Med 2001;52:1859–64.

60. Van Hoof E. The doctor-patient relationship in chronic fatigue syndrome: survey of patient perspectives. Qual Prim Care 2009;17:263–70.

61. Thomas MA, Smith AP. Primary healthcare provision and chronic fatigue syndrome: a survey of patients' and general practitioners' beliefs. BMC Fam Pract 2005;6:49.

62. Roberts AD, Charler ML, Papadopoulos A, et al. Does hypocortisolism predict a poor response to cognitive behavioural therapy in chronic fatigue syndrome? Psychol Med 2010;40:515–22.

63. Scheeres K, Wensing M, Bleijenberg G, et al. Implementing cognitive behavior therapy for chronic fatigue syndrome in mental health care: a costs and outcomes analysis. BMC Health Serv Res 2008;8:175.

64. Price JR, Mitchell E, Tidy E, et al. Cognitive behaviour therapy for chronic fatigue syndrome in adults. Cochrane Database Syst Rev 2008;3:CD001027.

65. Twisk FN, Maes M. A review on cognitive behavorial therapy (CBT) and graded exercise therapy (GET) in myalgic encephalomyelitis (ME)/chronic fatigue syndrome (CFS): CBT/GET is not only ineffective and not evidence-based, but also potentially harmful for many patients with ME/CFS. NeuroEndocrinol Lett 2009;30:284–99.

66. Wallman KE, Morton AR, Goodman C, et al. Randomised controlled trial of graded exercise in chronic fatigue syndrome. Med J Aust 2004;180:444–8.

67. Powell P, Bentall RP, Nye FJ, et al. Patient education to encourage graded exercise in chronic fatigue syndrome. 2-year follow-up of randomised controlled trial. Br J Psychiatry 2004;184:142–6.

68. Powell P, Bentall RP, Nye FJ, et al. Randomised controlled trial of patient education to encourage graded exercise in chronic fatigue syndrome. BMJ 2001;322:387–90.

69. White E. Erica White's beat candida cook book. Northamptonshire (UK): Thorson Publishers; 1999.

70. Hobday RA, Thomas S, O'Donovan A, et al. Dietary intervention in chronic fatigue syndrome. J Hum Nutr Diet 2008;21:141–9.

71. Baicus C, Baicus A. Spirulina did not ameliorate idiopathic chronic fatigue in four N-of-1 randomized controlled trials. Phytother Res. 2007;21:570–3.

72. Donaldson MS, Speight N, Loomis S, et al. Fibromyalgia syndrome improved using a mostly raw vegetarian diet: an observational study. BMC Complement Altern Med 2001;1:7.

73. Amsterdam JD, Shults J, Rutherford N. Open-label study of S-citalopram therapy of chronic fatigue syndrome and co-morbid major depressive disorder. Prog Neuropsychopharmacol Biol Psychiatry 2008;32:100–6.

74. Hartz AJ, Bentler SE, Brake KA, et al. The effectiveness of citalopram for idiopathic chronic fatigue. J Clin Psychiatry 2003;64:927–35.

75. Vercoulen JH, Swanink CM, Zitman FG, et al. Randomised, double-blind, placebo-controlled study of fluoxetine in chronic fatigue syndrome. Lancet 1996;347:858–61.

76. Heukeloma RO, Prinsb JB, Smitsa MG, et al. Influence of melatonin on fatigue severity in patients with chronic fatigue syndrome and late melatonin secretion. Eur J Neurol 2006;13:55–60.

77. Cox IM, Campbell MJ, Dowson D. Red blood cell magnesium and chronic fatigue syndrome. Lancet 1991;337:757–60.

78. Berbert AA, Kondo CR, Almendra CL, et al. Supplementation of fish oil and olive oil in patients with rheumatoid arthritis. Nutrition 2005;21:131–6.

79. Maes M, Mihaylova I, Leunis JC. In chronic fatigue syndrome, the decreased levels of omega-3 poly-unsaturated fatty acids are related to lowered serum zinc and defects in T cell activation. NeuroEndocrinol Lett 2005;26:745–51.

80. Behan PO, Behan WM. Essential fatty acids in the treatment of post-viral fatigue syndrome. In: Horrobin DF, editor. Omega-6 essential fatty acids: pathophysiology and roles in clinical medicine. New York: Wiley-Liss; 1990.

81. Behan PO, Behan WM, Horrobin D. Effect of high doses of essential fatty acids on the postviral fatigue syndrome. Acta Neurol Scand 1990;82:209–216, 272–82.

82. Warren G, McKendrick M, Peet M. The role of essential fatty acids in chronic fatigue syndrome. A case-controlled study of red-cell membrane essential fatty acids (EFA) and a placebo-controlled treatment study with high dose of EFA. Acta Neurol Scand 1999;99:112–6.

83. Mutch BJ, Banister EW. Ammonia metabolism in exercise and fatigue: a review. Med Sci Sport Exerc 1983;15:41–50.

84. Nybo L, Dalsgaard M, Steensberg A, et al. Cerebral ammonia uptake and accumulation during prolonged exercise in humans. J Physiol 2005;563 (Pt 1):285–90.

85. Sugino T, Shirai T, Kajimoto Y, et al. L-Ornithine supplementation attenuates physical fatigue in healthy volunteers by modulating lipid and amino acid metabolism. Nutr Res 2008;28:738–43.

86. Plioplys AV, Plioplys S. Amantadine and L-carnitine treatment of chronic fatigue syndrome. Neuropsychobiology 1997;35:16–23.

87. Tomassini V, Pozzilli C, Onesti E, et al. Comparison of the effects of acetyl L-carnitine and amantadine for the treatment of fatigue in multiple sclerosis: results of a pilot, randomised, double-blind, crossover trial. J Neurol Sci 2004;218:103–8.

88. Malaguarnera M, Gargante MP, Cristaldi E, et al. Acetyl L-carnitine (ALC) treatment in elderly patients with fatigue. Arch Gerontol Geriatr 2008;46:181–90.

89. Lloyd A, Hickie I, Wakefield D, et al. A double-blind, placebo-controlled trial of intravenous immunoglobulin therapy in patients with chronic fatigue syndrome. Am J Med 1990;89:561–8.

90. Vollmer-Conna U, Hickie I, Hadzi-Pavlovic D, et al. Intravenous immunoglobulin is ineffective in the treatment of patients with chronic fatigue syndrome. Am J Med 1997;103:38–43.

91. See DM, Tilles JG. Alpha-interferon treatment of patients with chronic fatigue syndrome. Immunol Invest 1996;25:153–64.

92. McKenzie R, O'Fallon A, Dale J, et al. Low-dose hydrocortisone for treatment of chronic fatigue syndrome: a randomized controlled trial, JAMA 1998;280:1061–6.

93. Cleare AJ, Heap E, Malhi GS, et al. Low-dose hydrocortisone in chronic fatigue syndrome: a randomised crossover trial. Lancet 1999;353:455–8.

94. Blockmans D, Persoons P, Van Houdenhove B, et al. Combination therapy with hydrocortisone and fludrocortisone does not improve symptoms in chronic fatigue syndrome: a randomized, placebo-controlled, double-blind, crossover study. Am J Med 2003;114:736–41.

95. Blockmans D, Persoons P, Van Houdenhove B, et al. Does methylphenidate reduce the symptoms of chronic fatigue syndrome? Am J Med 2006;119:167e23–30.

96. Olson LG, Ambrogetti A, Sutherland DC. A pilot randomized controlled trial of dexamphetamine in patients with chronic fatigue syndrome. Psychosomatics 2003; 44:38–43.

97. Randall DC, Cafferty FH, Shneerson JM, et al. Chronic treatment with modafinil may not be beneficial in patients with chronic fatigue syndrome. J Psychopharmacol 2005;19:647–60.

Toward a Comprehensive Differential Diagnosis and Clinical Approach to Fatigue in the Elderly

Vincent Morelli, MD

KEYWORDS
- Elderly • Fatigue • Causes • Differential diagnosis

Now that the definitions and treatments of recent, prolonged, chronic, and idiopathic fatigue have been presented, one must ask how useful these definitions are in clinical practice. Although it is important to know the data and definitions as presented, the arbitrary time frames of the definitions (1 month for recent fatigue, less than 6 months for prolonged fatigue, greater than 6 months for chronic fatigue) are less useful in the initial clinical setting.

Most clinicians, instead of concerning themselves with definitions, will instead start some type of workup as soon as a patient presents to the office. It is important to remember that two-thirds of patients with fatigue will have an identifiable cause that can be elucidated with a careful history and appropriate laboratory tests. This article aims to present primary care physicians with an encompassing approach to fatigue and to help generate a comprehensive differential diagnosis.

INFECTIOUS CAUSES

Viral infections are in the differential diagnosis of causes of fatigue. Hepatitis A, B, C, Epstein–Barr virus (EBV), human immunodeficiency virus (HIV), and retrovirus xeno-tropic murine leukemia related-virus (XMRV) are common causes of fatigue. In hepatitis A and B, up to 90% of infections are subclinical and, in hepatitis C, 60% to 70% of cases are subclinical.[1–3] With such subclinical disease, patients may present with mild nonspecific symptoms such as fatigue; thus, it is important to always check for hepatitis in fatigue patients.

In addition, although 95% of patients with mononucleosis present with fever, fatigue, pharyngitis, and lymphadenopathy, making the diagnosis fairly obvious, it should be remembered that fever, lymphadenopathy, and pharyngitis resolve within a

The author has nothing to disclose.
Department of Family and Community Medicine, Meharry Medical College, 1005 Dr D.B. Todd, Jr Boulevard Nashville, TN 37208, USA
E-mail address: vmorelli@mmc.edu

Clin Geriatr Med 27 (2011) 687–692
doi:10.1016/j.cger.2011.07.012
0749-0690/11/$ – see front matter © 2011 Elsevier Inc. All rights reserved.

month whereas fatigue usually persists for several months.[4] Therefore, it is important to keep mononucleosis on the differential diagnosis list.

The same holds true for HIV, wherein primary HIV usually presents with nonspecific flulike symptoms. Of note, neither Lyme disease nor secondary syphilis has been shown to be associated with isolated fatigue.

IMMUNE/RHEUMATOLOGIC CAUSES

Although fatigue is a common symptom in rheumatoid arthritis and systemic lupus erythematosus (SLE), fatigue as an *isolated* presenting complaint in these conditions is not documented in the literature. Still, because fatigue is such a prominent symptom and because an "insidious/general onset syndrome" (stiffness, fatigue, myalgia, low-grade fever) is well documented in rheumatoid arthritis,[5] these immune diseases should be kept in the differential diagnosis.

Celiac disease often presents as subclinical disease, often with fatigue, mood changes, or nonspecific symptoms.[6] Indeed, a high percentage of celiac disease is undiagnosed. In one screening study, a remarkable 7:1 ratio of undiagnosed to diagnosed celiac disease was found.[7] In addition, as many as 15% of newly diagnosed patients with celiac disease are older than 65 years and have nonspecific symptoms,[8] making it important to keep celiac disease in one's differential diagnosis.

Fibromyalgia should also be considered as a causative malady in fatigue, though the diagnosis of fibromyalgia is fairly obvious with its complaints of fatigue along with widespread pain and tenderness at 11 of 18 locations.

Similarly, polymyalgia rheumatica, presenting with fatigue in 40% of cases, is usually not hard to distinguish. The classic and telltale proximal muscle pain/stiffness/weakness is present in up to 95% of patients.[9]

ENDOCRINE CAUSES OF FATIGUE

Endocrine causes of fatigue include not only hypothyroidism but also subclinical hypothyroidism. Subclinical hypothyroidism with fatigue deserves a trial of low-dose thyroid hormone replacement therapy.

In addition, the primary care physician should remember that the most common symptom in peri-/postmenopausal patients is fatigue, present in more than 50% of patients.[10] Treatment in these cases may include exercise, testosterone, or hormone replacement.[11,12]

Another area of endocrine interest is growth hormone supplementation in aging patients who naturally experience age-related decline in growth hormone levels. Supplementation improved fatigue in several small studies.[13–16] However, side effects must be considered and long-term side effects in the elderly are unknown.

Androgen replacement for "andropause" has been shown to improve sexual function, lean body mass, bone density, and strength but has not yet been shown to be helpful in improving fatigue or increasing vigor.[17,18] Again, side effects must be considered.

In addition, the physician may consider adrenal insufficiency, especially in patients ending long-term steroid therapy and in those with mild congenital adrenal hyperplasia—which has been shown to occur more commonly than previously thought.[19]

NEOPLASTIC CAUSES FOR FATIGUE

Although the literature is replete with discussions of multifactorial fatigue in cancer patients, fatigue as a *presenting* complaint in cancer is *not* documented in the literature.

TOXINS

Toxins such as carbon monoxide should be considered. Carbon monoxide is produced by wood-burning stoves, kerosene heaters, automobile exhaust and coal burning plants. When carbon dioxide levels are high, symptoms such as headache, dizziness, and flulike symptoms are easier to pick up on. However, when chronic low-level exposure occurs, more subtle symptoms exist. Depression, fatigue, confusion, and memory loss are more common and make a toxic history vital to diagnosis.

Similarly, with exposure to heavy metals, acute high-level exposure is rather easy to diagnose whereas low-level chronic exposure is more difficult. Again, these must be uncovered by a detailed history. (For further information on toxins in the elderly, see the article by Dr Asma Jafri on aging and toxins in this issue.)

DIETARY FACTORS

Dietary indiscretions fall into the same category and should be sought out and addressed. Classic dietary problems such as the "tea and toast" diet of the elderly or in strict vegans may be contributory. In addition, overindulgences as well as malnourishment can also contribute to fatigue. A detailed dietary history should not be overlooked in the search for causative factors in fatigue.

Vitamin B_{12}

It is important to remember that subclinical vitamin B_{12} deficiency (from absorption problems, proton pump inhibitor [PPI] overuse, excessive alcohol, or "tea and toast" diets) can exist in the elderly and can result in fatigue, weight loss, neuropathy, memory impairment, or depression. In one study, 15% of adults older than 65 years were found to have evidence of vitamin B_{12} deficiency.[20] It is also important to note that up to 28% of patients can have normal hemoglobin and hematocrit (H/H),[21] mean corpuscular volume (MCV), and vitamin B_{12} levels as well. Screening for homocysteine and methylmalonic acid (MMA) levels is the preferred way to diagnose subclinical vitamin B_{12} deficiency in this population.

Vitamin D

A recent British survey found that more than 50% of adults have lower than normal vitamin D levels, and 16% had severe deficiency during winter months where exposure to sunshine was limited. In addition, many studies[22] have claimed that vitamin D deficiency affects systems other than the musculoskeletal system, such as cardiovascular,[23] respiratory,[24] neurologic,[25] neoplastic,[26,27] and has been associated with falls in the elderly.[28] A careful 2011 review by the Institute of Medicine[29] states that for extraskeletal outcomes, including cancer, cardiovascular disease, diabetes, and autoimmune disorders, the evidence is inconsistent, inconclusive, and generally uninformative.

However, a vitamin D deficient state *can* cause nonspecific symptoms such as fatigue, loss of muscle strength, bone and muscle pain, arthralgias, fibromyalgia-like syndromes, poor balance, and low mood.[30] Thus, symptoms consisting of muscle pains and weakness or fatigue may warrant a look into vitamin D levels.

The Institute of Medicine recommends 600 IU/day of vitamin D for people aged 1 to 70 years and 800 IU/day for those 71 years and older. Normal serum levels of 25-hydroxyvitamin D should be at least at least 20 ng/mL (50 nmol/liter).

MEDICATIONS

Although reviewing the myriad of medications that may contribute to fatigue is beyond the scope of this article, it should be obvious to the evaluating physician that medication imbalances need to be investigated and corrected.

SLEEP DISTURBANCES

Sleep disturbances caused by sleep apnea, jet lag, shift work, or increased life stress must also be considered because they obviously can contribute to fatigue. Proper sleep hygiene may prove helpful if no medical/psychological cause for sleep disturbances may be found.

CARDIOVASCULAR, PULMONARY, AND OTHER PHYSICAL DISEASES

Physical disease contributes significantly to fatigue and strong associations have been documented between chronic fatigue syndrome (CFS) and physical illness.[31] Physical illness should be accounted for in the evaluation of fatigue and, naturally, common cardiac/pulmonary conditions such as congestive heart failure (CHF) and chronic obstructive pulmonary disease (COPD) may be considered causative. Such conditions should be medically optimized in patients to minimize fatigue.

PSYCHIATRIC DISORDERS

Obviously, because there is such an overlap of fatigue and psychiatric conditions, one must consider psychological diagnoses when working up fatigue. However, although these conditions *may* be causative in fatigue, they are not necessarily so. A psychiatric diagnosis does not preclude a concomitant medical cause for fatigue or a diagnosis of CFS or idiopathic fatigue.

LABORATORY EVALUATIONS TO CONSIDER IN FATIGUE PATIENTS

Obviously no boiler-plate approach is useful with such a wide range of differential diagnoses to entertain. Some of the laboratory tests we consider in selected patients presenting with fatigue are the following:

- H/H
- Transferrin saturation
- Ferritin
- Thyroid-stimulating hormone (TSH)
- Growth hormone (GH)
- Testosterone
- Adrenocorticotropic hormone (ACTH) stimulation test
- Vitamin B_{12}/MMA
- Red blood cell magnesium
- Hepatitis panel
- Heterophile ab/EBV, IgM, IgG
- Primary HIV tests
- Primary tuberculosis (TB) tests
- Chest radiograph
- Erythrocyte sedimentation rate (ESR)
- C-reactive protein (CRP)
- Rheumatoid factor (RF)
- Antinuclear antibody (ANA)
- Celiac IgA antibodies to endomysium, endomysial antigen

- Tissue transglutaminase
- Lead/mercury/carboxyhemoglobin levels
- Cancer screening.

SUMMARY

The problem of fatigue in the elderly is more common than previously thought. The primary care physician must first inquire specifically about symptoms and then approach those with complaints with a broad differential diagnosis in mind and proceed in a systematic manner. The approach outlined in this article should help the geriatrician in this endeavor.

REFERENCES

1. Ayoola EA. Antibody to hepatitis a virus in healthy Nigerians. J Natl Med Assoc 1982;74:465–8.
2. Acorn CJ, Millar CC, Hoffman SK, et al. Viral hepatitis: a review. Optom Vis Sci 1995;72:763–9.
3. Wilkins T, Malcolm JK, Raina D, et al. Hepatitis C: diagnosis and treatment. Am Fam Physician 2010;81:1351–7.
4. Rea TD, Russo JE, Katon W, et al. Prospective study of the natural history of infectious mononucleosis caused by Epstein-Barr virus. J Am Board Fam Pract 2001;14:234–42.
5. Grassi W, De Angelis R, Lamanna G, et al. The clinical features of rheumatoid arthritis. Eur J Radiol 1998;27(Suppl 1):S18–24.
6. Bottaro G, Cataldo F, Rotolo N, et al. The clinical pattern of subclinical/silent celiac disease: an analysis on 1026 consecutive cases. Am J Gastroenterol 1999;94:691–6.
7. Catassi C, Fabiani E, Rätsch IM, et al. The coeliac iceberg in Italy. A multicentre antigliadin antibodies screening for coeliac disease in school-age subjects. Acta Paediatr Suppl 1996;412:29–35.
8. Patel D, Kalkat P, Baisch D, et al. Celiac disease in the elderly. Gerontology 2005;51: 213–4.
9. Brooks RC, McGee SR. Diagnostic dilemmas in polymyalgia rheumatica. Arch Intern Med 1997;157:162–8.
10. Bryant SE, Palav A, McCaffrey RJ. A review of symptoms commonly associated with menopause: implications for clinical neuropsychologists and other health care providers. Neuropsychol Rev 2003;13:145–52.
11. Daley A, MacArthur C, Mutrie N, et al. Exercise for vasomotor menopausal symptoms. Cochrane Database Syst Rev 2007;4:CD006108.
12. Somboonporn W. Testosterone therapy for postmenopausal women: efficacy and safety. Semin Reprod Med 2006;24:115–24.
13. McMillan CV, Bradley C, Gibney J, et al. Psychometric properties of two measures of psychological well-being in adult growth hormone deficiency. Health Qual Life Outcomes 2006;4:16.
14. Clayton P, Gleeson H, Monson J, et al. Growth hormone replacement throughout life: insights into age-related responses to treatment. Growth Horm IGF Res 2007;17: 369–82.
15. Koltowska-Haggstrom M, Mattsson AF, Monson JP, et al. Does long-term GH replacement therapy in hypopituitary adults with GH deficiency normalise quality of life? Eur J Endocrinol 2006;155:109–19.
16. Alexopoulou O, Abs R, Maiter D. Treatment of adult growth hormone deficiency: who, why and how? A review. Acta Clin Belg 2010;65:13–22.

17. Legros JJ, Meuleman EJ, Elbers JM, et al. Oral testosterone replacement in symptomatic late-onset hypogonadism: effects on rating scales and general safety in a randomized, placebo-controlled study. Eur J Endocrinol 2009;160:821–31.
18. Ly LP, Jimenez M, Zhuang TN, et al. A double-blind, placebo-controlled, randomized clinical trial of transdermal dihydrotestosterone gel on muscular strength, mobility, and quality of life in older men with partial androgen deficiency. J Clin Endocrinol Metab 2001;86:4078–88.
19. Deaton MA, Glorioso JE, McLean DB. Congenital adrenal hyperplasia: not really a zebra. Am Fam Physician 1999;59:1190–6, 1172.
20. Pennypacker LC, Allen RH, Kelly JP, et al. High prevalence of cobalamin deficiency in elderly outpatients. J Am Geriatr Soc 1992;40:1197–204.
21. Savage DG, Lindenbaum J, Stabler SP, et al. Sensitivity of serum methylmalonic acid and total homocysteine determinations for diagnosing cobalamin and folate deficiencies. Am J Med 1994;96:239–46.
22. Chu MP, Alagiakrishnan K, Sadowski C. The cure of ageing: vitamin D—magic or myth? Postgrad Med J 2010;86:608–16.
23. Ginde A, Scragg R, Schwartz RS, et al. Prospective study of serum 25-hydroxyvitamin D level, cardiovascular disease mortality, and all-cause mortality in older US adults. J Am Geriatr Soc 2009;57:1595–603.
24. Nurmatov U, Devereux G, Sheikh A. Nutrients and foods for the primary prevention of asthma and allergy: systematic review and meta-analysis. J Allergy Clin Immunol 2011;127:724–33.
25. Nimitphong H, Holick MF. Vitamin D, neurocognitive functioning and immunocompetence. Curr Opin Clin Nutr Metab Care 2011;14:7–14.
26. Yin L, Grandi N, Raum E, et al. Meta-analysis: longitudinal studies of serum vitamin D and colorectal cancer risk. Aliment Pharmacol Ther 2009;30:113–25.
27. Chen P, Hu P, Xie D, et al. Meta-analysis of vitamin D, calcium and the prevention of breast cancer. Breast Cancer Res Treat 2010;121:469–77.
28. Michael YL, Whitlock EP, Lin JS, et al. Primary care-relevant interventions to prevent falling in older adults: a systematic evidence review for the U.S. Preventive Services Task Force. Ann Intern Med 2010;153:815–25.
29. Ross AC, Manson JE, Abrams SA, et al. The 2011 report on dietary reference intakes for calcium and vitamin d from the institute of medicine: what clinicians need to know. J Clin Endocrinol Metab 2011;96:53–8.
30. Sievenpiper JL, McIntyre EA, Verrill M, et al. Unrecognised severe vitamin D deficiency. BMJ 2008;336:1371–4.
31. Resnick HE, Carter EA, Aloia M, et al. Cross-sectional relationship of reported fatigue to obesity, diet, and physical activity: results from the third national health and nutrition examination survey. J Clin Sleep Med 2006;2:163–9.

Index

Note: Page numbers of article titles are in **boldface** type.

A

Abdominal aortic aneurysm, 528
Abuse and neglect, prevention of, 534
Aging, and disease prevention, **523–539**
  and effects of vitamins and supplements, **591–607**
  and toxins, **609–628**
  as inevitable process, 508
  attitudes about, 646–648
  autoimmune theory of, 495
  cellular and functional changes of, 492–494
  cellular senescence theory of, 510
  chromosomal alterations and, 495
  coping and, 652–653
  developmental-genetic theory of, 495
  emotional well-being in, 652
  exercise and, 514–515, 524–525, **661–671**
    special considerations for, 666–667
  extracellular mechanisms of, 631–632
  free radial theory of, 510–511
  glycation theory of, 511
  healthy behavior in, 523–525
  metabolic disorders in, 525–527
  myths and realities of, 646, 647
  neuroendocrinologic theory of, 495
  organ system mechanisms of, 496
  personality and, 651–652
  primacy of mitochondrial decay in, 511
  psychological factors in, **645–660**
  religiosity and spirituality and, 653–654
  self-perceptions concerning, 648
  sexual relationships in, 650–651
  social relationships in, 648–651
  social support in, 649–650
  successful, definition of, 577
    optimal diet for, 583
  successful versus usual, 502–503
  telemere theory of, 495
  theories of, 491–495, 510–511
    and mechanisms of, **491–505**
  theory of oxidative stress and, 491–495

Clin Geriatr Med 27 (2011) 693–699
doi:10.1016/S0749-0690(11)00073-5
0749-0690/11/$ – see front matter © 2011 Elsevier Inc. All rights reserved.

geriatric.theclinics.com

Air pollution, 609–612
  indoor, 609–612
  outdoor, 609–612
Alcohol, 612–613
Alcohol dehydrogenase, 613
Alzheimer's disease, biomarkers of, 635–636
    dementia in, 634
    prevention of amyloid plaque formation in, 636
    removal of Aß-amyloid protein from brain in, 637
    treatment and prevention of, 636
Anti-aging clinics, 516
Anti-aging medicines, 508, 509
Anti-aging trends, pharmaceutical industry and, 507
    state of art in, **507–522**
Antidepressants, in chronic fatigue, 678–679
Antioxidants, 591–592

B

B vitamins, and cancer, 595
  and dementia, 594–595
  and folic acid, 594–596
  and vascular disease, 594
Balance and gait, in aging, 496
Benzodiazepines, 617
Beta carotene(s), and cancer, 592
  macular degeneration and, 592
Bioidentical hormones, 544–546
  large scale studies of, 547–548
  versus synthetic, 544, 545
Body structure and composition, with aging, 496
Brain, aging, and neurodegenerative diseases, **629–644**
  changes in, with aging and disease, 630
  external factors and, 630–631
Brain cells, cell death and, 631
Breast cancer, 529–530
  bioidentical progesterone versus synthetic progestins in, 546–547

C

Calcium, 599–600
Caloric restriction, in aging, 512–514, 582–583
Cancer(s), B vitamins and, 595
  beta carotenes and, 592
  in older adults, 528–530
Cardiovascular disease, 527–528
Cardiovascular events, bioidentical progesterone versus synthetic progestins
    in, 548
Cardiovascular risk, and estrogen, 548
Cardiovascular system, in aging, 498–499
Carotenoids, vitamin A and, 592

Cell death, brain cells and, 631
Cerebrovascular disease, 527
Cervical cancer, 529
Chemical exposure, 622
Chronic fatigue syndrome, clinical manifestations of, 675
  definition of, 673–674
  factors predisposing to, 676
  precipitating and perpetuating factors in, 676–677
  primary care approach to, 676
  prognosis in, 677
  treatment of, 677–681
Chronic obstructive pulmonary disease, exercise in, 666
Cigarette smoking, 612
Cognitive decline, vitamin E and, 593
Cold exposure, and hypothermia, 614–616
Colorectal cancer, 528–529
Congestive heart failure, exercise and, 666–667
Coronary heart disease, 527
Corticosteroids, in chronic fatigue, 680
Cortisol levels, exercise and, 514

D

Dehydroepiandrosterone, 517–518, 600
Dementia, B vitamins and, 594–595
  cognitive activity and, 639
  dietary alterations and, 638
  exercise and, 666
  hormone replacement and, 639
  physical activity and, 639
  risk factors and prevention of, 637–640
Dental changes, in aging, 497
Depression, 531
Diabetes mellitus, 525–526
Dietary factors, fatigue and, 678, 689
Dietary patterns, and aging, 578–583
Diet(s), alterations in, dementia and, 638
  for successful aging, **577–589**
  high protein low carbohydrate, 581–582
  Mediterranean. See Mediterranean diet.
  of centenarians, Okinawa diet, 580–581
  optimal, for successful aging, 583
  vegetarian, 581
  Western, 578–579
Disease, prevention of, aging and, **523–539**
Drinking water, 618–621
  chemicals in, regulation by EPA, 619
  microbial agents in, regulation by EPA, 619
Driver safety, 533

E

Environmental temperature exposures, 614–616
Estrogen, and cardiovascular risk, 548
    and progesterone, 542–544
        current recommendations on, 543–544
        making decision on, 543
        Women's Health Initiative and, 542–543
Exercise, and osteoarthritis, 666
    barriers to, 662
    benefits of, 661–662
    comorbidities and, 663
    dementia and, 666
    in aging, 514–515, 524–525, **661–671**
    preparticipation screening for, 663–664
    safety concerns and, 662–663
    tools to motivate, 663
Exercise prescription, 664–666

F

Fatigue, and chronic fatigue, in elderly, **673–686**
    chronic, prevalence of, 674–675
    dietary factors and, 678, 689
    endocrine causes of, 688
    immune/rheumatologic causes of, 688
    in elderly, clinical approach to, comprehensive differential diagnosis and, **687–692**
    infectious causes of, 687–688
    laboratory evaluations in, 690–691
    neoplastic causes for, 688–689
    normal, with aging, 675
    sleep disturbances and, 690
    toxins as cause of, 689
Folic acid, B vitamins and, 594–596

G

Gastrointestinal system, in aging, 500
Ginkgo biloba, 600–601

H

Hearing, in aging, 497, 532
Heat exposure, 614
Hematopoietic system, in aging, 502
Herbal medications, 617–618
Herpes zoster (Shingles), 530
Hormone preparations, in women, state of evidence of, 544–546
Hormone replacement, dementia and, 639
Hormone replacement therapy, in geriatric patient, **541–559, 561–575**
Human growth hormone, 516–517
Hyperlipidemia, 526

Hypertension, 527–528
  exercise and, 667
Hypothermia, cold exposure and, 614–616
Hypothyroidism, 527
  diagnosis of, 567–569
  symptoms of, 567
  treatment of, 569–570

I

Immunizations, for older adults, 530–531
Immunotherapy, in chronic fatigue, 680
Incontinence, 533
Influenza, 530
Insulin, exercise and, 515
Integumentary system changes, in aging, 496–497

L

Lifestyle, ideal and poor, vitality between, compared, 510

M

Macular degeneration, beta carotenes and, 592
Mediterranean diet, 579–580
  and ARCD, 580
  and cancer, 580
  cardioprotective effects of, 579–580
Mental health, of older adults, 531
Metabolic disorders, in aging, 525–527
Metformin, 514
  and vitamin B_{12}, 595–596
Mitochondrial dysfunction, 632
Musculoskeletal problems, 531
Musculoskeletal system, in aging, 498

N

National Institute of Health conference report, on prevention of cognitive decline,
  639–640
Nervous system, in aging, 501–502
Neurodegenerative diseases, aging brain and, **629–644**
Neuroendocrine system, and autoregulation, in aging, 502
Nonsteroidal anti-inflammatory drugs (NSAIDs), 616–617
Nutrition, 524

O

Omega-3 fatty acids, 601
Osteoarthritis, exercise and, 666
Osteoporosis, 531–532
  vitamin A and, 592
Over-the-counter (OTC) medications, 617

P

Parkinson's disease, clinical diagnosis of, 633
  neuroimaging in, 633–634
  pathogenesis of, 634
  symptoms of, 632–633
Personality, and aging, 651–652
Pneumococcal infection, 530–531
Polypharmacy, avoiding effects from, 534
Prescription drugs, 616–617
Progesterone. See also *Estrogen, and progesterone.*
  bioidentical, versus synthetic progestins, 546
Prostate cancer, 529
Proteinopathies, 631
Psychological factors, in aging, **645–660**
Pulmonary system, in aging, 499–500

R

Radiation, 621–622
Rapamycin, 513
Religiosity and spirituality, aging and, 653–654
Renal system, in aging, 500–501
Resveratrol, 512–513

S

Secondhand smoke, 612
Selenium, 594
SENS strategy, 515–516
Sexual relationships, in aging, 650–651
Sleep, for older adults, 525
Social relationships, in aging, 648–651
Socioemotional selectivity theory, 648–649
Stimulants, in chronic fatigue, 681
Supplements, and vitamins, effects on aging, **591–607**
  in chronic fatigue, 679–680

T

Taste, sensitivity of, in aging, 497–498
Testosterone, 517
  decline with aging, 562
  for women, 548–550
    risks of, 549
    therapeutic trials of, 550
  low serum, effects of, 562
  physiologic effects of, 561–562
  supplementation, cardiovascular benefits of, 563
    cognitive function and, 564
    effects of, 563–565
    in depression, 564

in frailty, 563–564
  potential side effects of, 565–567
  sexual function and, 565
Tobacco cessation, 523–524
Toxins, and aging, **609–628**
  as cause of fatigue, 689

U

Urogenital system, in aging, 501

V

Vascular disease, B vitamins and, 594
  vitamin E and, 593
Vegetarian diet, 581
Vision acuity, in aging, 497, 533
Vitamin A, and carotenoids, 592
  and osteoporosis, 592
Vitamin B$_{12}$, deficiency of, 595, 689
  sources of, 595
Vitamin D, cancer prevention and, 597
  cardiovascular disease and, 598
  current intake of, 596
  deficiency of, 597, 689
  falls and, 597
  fracture prevention and, 597
  normal serum levels of, 596–597
  physiology of, 596
  safety of, 598
  supplementation, 598–599
Vitamin E, and cognitive decline, 593
  vascular disease and, 593
Vitamin K, 600
Vitamins, and supplements, effects on aging, **591–607**

W

Western diet, 578–579

United States Postal Service

Statement of Ownership, Management, and Circulation
(All Periodicals Publications Except Requestor Publications)

1. Publication Title	2. Publication Number								3. Filing Date
Clinics in Geriatric Medicine	0	0	0	-	7	0	4		9/16/11

4. Issue Frequency	5. Number of Issues Published Annually	6. Annual Subscription Price
Feb, May, Aug, Nov	4	$241.00

7. Complete Mailing Address of Known Office of Publication (Not printer) (Street, city, county, state, and ZIP+4®)

Elsevier Inc.
360 Park Avenue South
New York, NY 10010-1710

Contact Person
Amy S. Beacham

Telephone (Include area code)
215-239-3687

8. Complete Mailing Address of Headquarters or General Business Office of Publisher (Not printer)

Elsevier Inc., 360 Park Avenue South, New York, NY 10010-1710

9. Full Names and Complete Mailing Addresses of Publisher, Editor, and Managing Editor (Do not leave blank)

Publisher (Name and complete mailing address)

Kim Murphy, Elsevier, Inc., 1600 John F. Kennedy Blvd. Suite 1800, Philadelphia, PA 19103-2899

Editor (Name and complete mailing address)

Yonah Korngold, Elsevier, Inc., 1600 John F. Kennedy Blvd. Suite 1800, Philadelphia, PA 19103-2899

Managing Editor (Name and complete mailing address)

Barton Dudlick, Elsevier, Inc., 1600 John F. Kennedy Blvd. Suite 1800, Philadelphia, PA 19103-2899

10. Owner (Do not leave blank. If the publication is owned by a corporation, give the name and address of the corporation immediately followed by the names and addresses of all stockholders owning or holding 1 percent or more of the total amount of stock. If not owned by a corporation, give the names and addresses of the individual owners. If owned by a partnership or other unincorporated firm, give its name and address as well as those of each individual owner. If the publication is published by a nonprofit organization, give its name and address.)

Full Name	Complete Mailing Address
Wholly owned subsidiary of	4520 East-West Highway
Reed/Elsevier, US holdings	Bethesda, MD 20814

11. Known Bondholders, Mortgagees, and Other Security Holders Owning or Holding 1 Percent or More of Total Amount of Bonds, Mortgages, or Other Securities. If none, check box. ☐ None

Full Name	Complete Mailing Address
N/A	

12. Tax Status (For completion by nonprofit organizations authorized to mail at nonprofit rates) (Check one)
The purpose, function, and nonprofit status of this organization and the exempt status for federal income tax purposes:
☐ Has Not Changed During Preceding 12 Months
☐ Has Changed During Preceding 12 Months (Publisher must submit explanation of change with this statement)

PS Form 3526, September 2007 (Page 1 of 3 (Instructions Page 3)) PSN 7530-01-000-9931 PRIVACY NOTICE: See our Privacy policy in www.usps.com

---

13. Publication Title	14. Issue Date for Circulation Data Below
Clinics in Geriatric Medicine	August 2011

15. Extent and Nature of Circulation		Average No. Copies Each Issue During Preceding 12 Months	No. Copies of Single Issue Published Nearest to Filing Date
a. Total Number of Copies (Net press run)		940	748
b. Paid Circulation (By Mail and Outside the Mail)	(1) Mailed Outside-County Paid Subscriptions Stated on PS Form 3541. (Include paid distribution above nominal rate, advertiser's proof copies, and exchange copies)	426	386
	(2) Mailed In-County Paid Subscriptions Stated on PS Form 3541 (Include paid distribution above nominal rate, advertiser's proof copies, and exchange copies)		
	(3) Paid Distribution Outside the Mails Including Sales Through Dealers and Carriers, Street Vendors, Counter Sales, and Other Paid Distribution Outside USPS®	164	164
	(4) Paid Distribution by Other Classes Mailed Through the USPS (e.g. First-Class Mail®)		
c. Total Paid Distribution (Sum of 15b (1), (2), (3), and (4))	▶	590	550
d. Free or Nominal Rate Distribution (By Mail and Outside the Mail)	(1) Free or Nominal Rate Outside-County Copies Included on PS Form 3541	56	63
	(2) Free or Nominal Rate In-County Copies Included on PS Form 3541		
	(3) Free or Nominal Rate Copies Mailed at Other Classes Through the USPS (e.g. First-Class Mail)		
	(4) Free or Nominal Rate Distribution Outside the Mail (Carriers or other means)		
e. Total Free or Nominal Rate Distribution (Sum of 15d (1), (2), (3) and (4))	▶	56	63
f. Total Distribution (Sum of 15c and 15e)	▶	646	613
g. Copies not Distributed (See instructions to publishers #4 (page #3))	▶	294	135
h. Total (Sum of 15f and g)	▶	940	746
i. Percent Paid (15c divided by 15f times 100)		91.33%	89.72%

16. Publication of Statement of Ownership

☐ If the publication is a general publication, publication of this statement is required. Will be printed in the November 2011 issue of this publication.

☐ Publication not required.

17. Signature and Title of Editor, Publisher, Business Manager, or Owner		Date
[signature] Amy S. Beacham – Senior Inventory Distribution Coordinator		September 16, 2011

I certify that all information furnished on this form is true and complete. I understand that anyone who furnishes false or misleading information on this form or who omits material or information requested on the form may be subject to criminal sanctions (including fines and imprisonment) and/or civil sanctions (including civil penalties).

PS Form 3526, September 2007 (Page 2 of 3)

Moving?

Make sure your subscription moves with you!

To notify us of your new address, find your **Clinics Account Number** (located on your mailing label above your name), and contact customer service at:

Email: journalscustomerservice-usa@elsevier.com

800-654-2452 (subscribers in the U.S. & Canada)
314-447-8871 (subscribers outside of the U.S. & Canada)

Fax number: 314-447-8029

Elsevier Health Sciences Division
Subscription Customer Service
3251 Riverport Lane
Maryland Heights, MO 63043

*To ensure uninterrupted delivery of your subscription,
please notify us at least 4 weeks in advance of move.

Printed and bound by CPI Group (UK) Ltd, Croydon, CR0 4YY

03/10/2024

01040452-0003